Recent Advances, New Perspectives and Applications in the Treatment of Ovarian Cancer

Edited by Michael Friedrich

Published in London, United Kingdom

Recent Advances, New Perspectives and Applications in the Treatment of Ovarian Cancer
http://dx.doi.org/10.5772/intechopen.100847
Edited by Michael Friedrich

Contributors
Nicola Di Santo, Greta Bagnolini, Yin Wong, Marco Carnelli, Luigi Frigerio, Mustafa Kemal Ruhi, Imran Rizvi, Brittany P. Rickard, William J. Polacheck, Christos Valavanis, Efthymia Souka, Gabriela-Monica Stanc, Imam Malik Kabir, Abdulaziz Tahir Idris, Amar Ranjan, Lawanya Ranjan, Mansi Modi, Saransh Verma, Harshita Dubey, Ruchi Sinha, Harsh Goel, Pranay Tanwar, Ekta Rahul, Anita Chopra, Rani Kumari Mahkam, Neeraj Verma, Devender Singh Chauhan, Utkarsh Dubey

First published in London, United Kingdom, 2023 by IntechOpen
IntechOpen is the global imprint of INTECHOPEN LIMITED, registered in England and Wales, registration number: 11086078, 5 Princes Gate Court, London, SW7 2QJ, United Kingdom

British Library Cataloguing-in-Publication Data
A catalogue record for this book is available from the British Library

Additional hard and PDF copies can be obtained from orders@intechopen.com

Recent Advances, New Perspectives and Applications in the Treatment of Ovarian Cancer
Edited by Michael Friedrich
p. cm.
Print ISBN 978-1-80356-518-7
Online ISBN 978-1-80356-519-4
eBook (PDF) ISBN 978-1-80356-520-0

Meet the editor

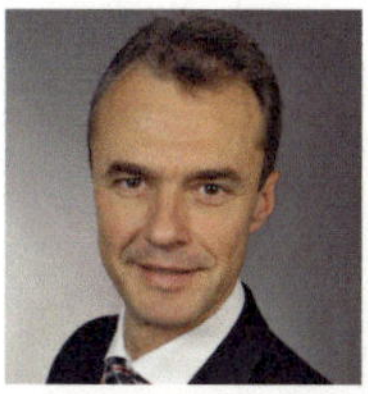

Michael Friedrich is a senior gynecological oncologist and oncological surgeon at Helios Klinikum Krefeld, Germany, and specializes in treating women with breast cancer and gynecological malignancies. He is a certified breast surgeon and has an academic appointment as an Associate Professor at the University of Schleswig-Holstein. He has received several awards for his scientific work, which focuses on vitamin D metabolism in gynecologic malignancies and the interaction of DNA-mismatch repair and resistance to chemotherapy. Further research interests are interstitial brachytherapy for recurrences of cervical cancer, the use of innovative therapies in gynecological malignancies, the sentinel lymph node technique in gynecological malignancies, especially in vulvar cancer, and the use of intraoperative intraperitoneal chemotherapy (HIPEC) in ovarian cancer. He is a member of several prestigious editorial and scientific boards and a member of Germany's committees for S3-guidelines for cervical, endometrial, vulvar and breast cancer. He is also a member of the Ethics Committee of the Nordrhein-Westphalen Medical Chamber, of the Board of directors of the BLFG (*Bundesarbeitsgemeinschaft leitender Frauenärzte*), of the Board of the German Society for Gynecology responsible for developing the continuous medical education curriculum in gynecology, and of the Society of Pelvic Surgeons.

Contents

Preface

Ovarian cancer is a heterogeneous disease composed of multiple distinct molecular and clinical subtypes. Improvements in the ability to target the underlying drivers of ovarian cancer, combined with advances in surgical techniques, are crucial for developing effective treatments for patients with ovarian cancer. In this book different aspects of recent advances, new perspectives and applications in the treatment of ovarian cancer will be addressed.

Several studies have been carried out to determine the complexity of ovarian cancer as a disease with multiple distinct types that presents with symptoms similar to those in other gynecological, gastrointestinal and genitourinary diseases. Most ovarian tumors are malignant variants of common epithelial and germ cell tumors, and are classified histologically based on the presumed tissue of origin. The first chapter is focusing on "A Succinct Molecular Profile of High-Grade Ovarian Cancer". Molecular diagnosis is now aiding the early detection and treatment of ovarian cancer even before metastasis sets in. Thus, studying the molecular profiles of each type is key to understanding the origin and pathogenesis as well as genetic aberrations and mutations involved in the development of the disease. Ovarian cancers originate either from the ovary or fallopian tube, and are principally found to harbor mutations in PTEN, KRAS, BRAF, BRCA1, BRCA2 and TP53, with TP53 mutations being the most frequent. Advanced methods of detecting these genes in blood and uterine lavage can be anticipated in the very near future. There is an urgent need for further studies on the detailed mechanisms underlying the role of mutant TP53 in ovarian cancer development and its potential role in therapeutic interventions.

Ovarian tumors are a heterogeneous group of neoplasms classified based on histopathologic type and grade of differentiation. They comprise a broad range of tumors from benign and borderline to malignant histotypes characterized by different histopathological, immunophenotypic and molecular features. The chapter "Recent Advances in Classification and Histopathological Diagnosis of Ovarian Epithelial Malignant Tumours" presents an overview of recent advances in ovarian epithelial malignant tumor classification along with the histopathological, immunophenotypic and molecular diagnostic criteria, highlighting discrepancies or changes in terminology, and diagnostic challenges. These changes provide a better understanding of the nature of ovarian tumors and lead to more efficient therapeutic management of these pathological entities.

The chapter "Role of Human Epididymis Protein 4 in Tumour Angiogenesis" discusses the human epididymis protein 4 (HE4), a secretory protein expressed in the reproductive tract and respiratory epithelium in normal individuals. The HE4 serum level is raised in various solid cancers, enabling its use as a diagnostic and prognostic biomarker. It is an established biomarker of epithelial ovarian cancer (EOC) and is also significant in various other malignancies including cancer of the endometrium, cervix, lung and breast. Studies also show HE4 as an independent prognostic biomarker in non-small cell lung carcinoma. HE4 promotes angiogenesis via the STAT3 signaling pathway.

The chapter "Integrins in Ovarian Cancer: Survival Pathways, Malignant Ascites and Targeted Photochemistry" describes the role of integrins in ovarian cancer. Integrins are surface adhesion molecules that, upon binding to ligands, cluster to form adhesion complexes. These adhesion complexes are comprised of structural and regulatory proteins that modulate a variety of cellular behaviors, including differentiation, growth, and migration, through bidirectional signaling activities. Aberrant integrin expression and activation in ovarian cancer play a key role in the detachment of cancer cells from primary sites as well as migration, invasion and spheroid formation. An emerging area is the activation or rearrangement of integrins due to mechanical stress in the tumor microenvironment, particularly in response to fluid shear stress imparted by currents of malignant ascites. The chapter focuses on the effect of malignant ascites and crosstalk with survival pathways, and reviews the literature on integrin-targeting approaches in ovarian cancer, including targeted photochemistry for therapy and imaging.

Epithelial ovarian cancer (EOC), the most lethal gynecologic malignancy in the Western world, has historically been treated with surgery followed by chemotherapy. The chapter "PARP Inhibitors in the Treatment of Epithelial Ovarian Cancer" examines the antineoplastic activity of poly (ADP-ribose) polymerase inhibitors (PARPis), one of the most active new targeted therapies for the treatment of EOC. PARPis' mechanism of action relies on their ability to interfere with DNA repair events, leading ultimately to cell death, the biological concept known as synthetic lethality. Initially developed as a maintenance therapy in patients responding to platinum-based chemotherapy in a recurrent setting, PARPis are now approved as a frontline treatment strategy. The chapter describes the clinical development studies which led to their approval, as well as safety and the management of adverse events associated with this new class of drugs. Rational considerations for the use of PARPis in the frontline setting are also discussed.

In summary, this book brings together a number of leading opinions and discoveries from experts treating ovarian cancer, highlighting the rapidly evolving understanding of the tumor biology of this devastating disease.

Michael Friedrich
Department of Obstetrics and Gynecology,
Helios Hospital,
Krefeld, Germany

Section 1

Molcular Profile and Classification of Ovarian Cancer

Chapter 1

A Succinct Molecular Profile of High-Grade Ovarian Cancer

Imam Malik Kabir and Abdulaziz Tahir Idris

Abstract

Several studies have been carried out to determine the complexity of ovarian cancer as a disease with multiple distinct types that presents with symptoms similar to those in other gynaecological, gastrointestinal and genitourinary diseases. The malignant variants of common epithelial and germ cell tumours constitute the bulk of ovarian tumours and are classified histologically based on the presumed tissue of origin. Molecular diagnosis is now aiding in the early detection and treatment of ovarian cancer even before metastasis sets in. Thus studying the molecular profiles of each type is key to understanding the origin and pathogenesis as well as genetic aberrations and mutations involved in the development of the disease. Ovarian cancers originate either from the ovary or fallopian tube and are found majorly to harbour mutations in *PTEN, KRAS, BRAF, BRCA1, BRCA2* and *TP53,* with *TP53* mutations being the most frequent. Genetic testing for ovarian cancers involves testing for the aforementioned genes, and in the nearest future, an advanced method that would detect these genes in blood and uterine lavage is expected. There is an urgent need for further studies on the detailed mechanisms underlying the roles of mutant *TP53* in ovarian cancer development and its potential role in therapeutic interventions.

Keywords: molecular profile, epithelial ovarian carcinoma, high-grade serous ovarian carcinoma, recurrent clear cell carcinoma, *TP53* mutations

1. Introduction

Ovarian Cancer is the eighth most common cancer among women worldwide, with an incidence of about 239,000 new cases and 152,000 deaths annually [1]. It is a complex disease with multiple distinct molecular and histologic types, each with different aetiology, risk factors, prognosis and response to treatment. Several factors make ovarian cancer treatment difficult, even though most patients experience or present symptoms, but such symptoms tend to overlap or mimic other symptoms presented in other gynaecological, genitourinary and gastrointestinal diseases. Therefore, early diagnosis is rarely achieved and as such, it is mostly carried out after metastasis [2].

Almost all malignant and benign ovarian tumours are of epithelial, stromal or germ cell origin, with those of epithelial origin accounting for more than 90% [3]. Malignant ovarian cancers also referred to as carcinomas are classified into five main histologic types (histotypes) namely: endometroid, mucinous, clear cell, low-grade serous and

Histologic Type	Features
High-grade Serous Ovarian carcinoma	• Tumour cells are atypical, with large irregular nuclei • Papillary growth pattern • Highly proliferative and aggressive • Targeted genes: *BRCA1* and *BRCA2*, and *TP53*
Low-grade Serous Ovarian carcinoma	• Tumour cells possess small uniform nuclei • Micro-papillary growth pattern • Low proliferative and less aggressive • Targeted genes: *KRAS, NRAS, BRAF*, and *PIK3CA*
Endometrioid	• Shows cystic and solid patterns • Usually associated with endometriosis • High grade have similar profile with HGSOC • Targeted genes: *ARID1A, POLE, PIK3CA, and PTEN*
Mucinous	• Large tumour cells filled with mucus-like substance • Early diagnosis • Targeted genes: *PIK3CA, HER2,and KRAS*
Clear cell	• Cells with clear cytoplasm containing glycogen • Papillary, solid, tubulo-cystic or mixed patterns of growth • Usually associated with endometriosis • Early diagnosis • Targeted genes: *ARID1A, PTEN*, and *PIK3CA,*

Table 1.
Salient features of histological subtypes of epithelial ovarian carcinomas.

high-grade serous ovarian carcinoma (**Table 1**). The pathogenesis and origin of ovarian cancer are not well understood. However, most tumours appear to originate from other parts of the reproductive system and affect the ovary secondarily [4].

One of the most common genetic abnormality seen in ovarian cancer is mutation and loss of *TP53* function, including DNA copy number abnormalities which affects cell proliferation and apoptosis [2].

Despite the continuous effort to develop early screening strategies, only a negligible fraction of ovarian cancers are diagnosed while they are localized to the ovaries. Diagnosis is mostly made after the disease has spread to the pelvic organs, abdomen, and/or beyond the peritoneal cavity, and this makes treatment difficult.

The standard treatment of ovarian cancer is platinum and taxane-based combination chemotherapy after cytoreductive surgery to remove a significant bulk of the tumour. Despite being considered chemosensitive, the majority of the patients subjected to cytoreductive surgery and combination therapy will need second-line chemotherapy due to tumour recurrence within 2 years [5].

2. Description of molecular profiles

Recently, ovarian cancers have been classified into type 1 and type 2 tumours. Type 1 constitutes of low-grade tumours (mucinous, endometrioid, low-grade serous and clear cell types) that harbour mutations in *PTEN, KRAS* and *BRAF* with microsatellite instability and are thought to originate from the ovary. While type 2 tumours are high-grade serous and carcinosarcomas that originate from the fallopian tube and have mutations in *BRCA1, BRCA2* and *TP53* [6–8].

Whole-exome and Whole-genome sequencing studies of ovarian cancer have not only revealed its genetic heterogeneity, but have identified the genomic effect of aberrant DNA damage and repair processes in endometrioid, high-grade serous, and clear cell ovarian cancers [9].

3. Histopathology of ovarian cancer

Ovarian tumours have different histologic features and patterns due to the different tissues found within the ovary. With increased histologic examinations over the years, the classification of ovarian tumours has evolved, which is mostly based on the presumed tissue of origin, and includes common epithelial tumours, lipoid cell tumours, gonadoblastoma, sex cord-stromal tumours, germ cell tumours, soft tissue tumours not specific to the ovary, metastatic tumours and unclassified tumours [10]. The malignant variants of the common epithelial tumours and germ cell tumours will be discussed briefly.

3.1 Common epithelial Tumours

Most benign and malignant ovarian tumours belong to this group and are derived from the common celomic epithelium on the surface of the ovary, which is also derived from the split lateral mesoderm and which also infolds to form the Mullerian duct. The Mullerian duct forms the endocervix, uterine corpus and uterine tube, thus explaining the different epithelial patterns (serous, mucinous, clear cell and endometrioid) in this group of tumours. Each of these patterns includes a completely benign (partly cystic, regular lining cells often covering stromal projections and with gland like spaces) type and an adenocarcinoma (with invasive features that are either well differentiated with gland-like spaces or poorly differentiated sheets). Between these two patterns is an intermediate pattern termed carcinoma of low malignant potential that exhibits cellular stratification with variable mitotic activity and clear atypia but without stromal invasion [10].

Histologic diagnosis of an ovarian tumour should be done on the primary tumour, not on the histologic pattern of metastasis because not all peritoneal lesions are metastases even when there is a confirmed primary ovarian carcinoma [11].

One of the problems associated with adenocarcinoma of low malignant potential and sometimes with low-grade adenocarcinoma is the evaluation of glandular structures in lymph nodes to determine if such are metastases or simple benign glandular inclusions. It is also vital to ascertain the significance of glandular inclusions in lymph nodes after surgical removal because the epithelium in benign inclusion is tubal with cilia, shows a simple papillary pattern and has peripheral gland-like spaces that may extend around lymphoid follicles and sometimes extends into a follicle, but without stromal response, while adenocarcinoma usually invades a follicle and often shows a desmoplastic response. Mitoses are rarely seen in benign inclusions but present in adenocarcinoma [10].

Invasion of stroma by cribriform-like tumour composed of strands of infiltrating malignant cells is a feature of mucinous adenocarcinoma. Mucinous tumours might either be of the endocervical or intestinal type, the former is characterized by cells with basal nuclei and the latter is characterized by goblet cells, sometimes argentaffin cells and rarely Paneth cells [10].

Clear cell carcinoma of the ovary usually arises from the ovarian surface epithelium, and sometimes from endometriosis and is said to represent a separate clinicopathologic entity. This carcinoma has been reported to exist in three architectural patterns viz.: solid, papillary and tubulocystic [12, 13]. Clear cell tumours are generally considered malignant due to failure to recognize benign or borderline types. Recent studies have found benign, borderline and micro-invasive tumours, with borderline tumours having 1–3 layers of clear, eosinophilic or hobnail cells, while the micro-invasive tumours showed evidence of focal stromal reaction with rare mitoses [14].

Endometrioid adenocarcinoma however is less common than the mucinous or serous type and has a histologic pattern similar to that of carcinoma of the endometrium that ranges from a well-differentiated glandular pattern to poorly differentiated adenocarcinoma with very few glands.

3.2 Malignant germ cell tumours

These are derived from the primitive germ cells found between the junction of the hindgut and yolk sac. They later migrate through the mesentery to the posterior wall of the embryo, just beneath the celomic epithelium. In the process of their migration, some germ cells become arrested or extend beyond their usual position to form extragonadal germ cell tumours that are histologically similar to those in the ovary. Most types of germ cell tumours occur in pure form, with few occurring in mixed form. Thus, multiple sections must be examined to make a definitive diagnosis.

Malignant germ tumours include dysgerminoma, endodermal sinus tumour, immature teratoma and mixed germ cell tumour. Dysgerminoma is similar to seminoma of the testis and is derived from undifferentiated germ cells, and consists of strands, sheets, and groups of cells that are large and uniform in size with a central nucleus and varying mitotic activity. Lymphoid follicles with germinal centres are sometimes present with some showing granulomatous reaction [10].

Endodermal sinus tumours exhibit a central vascular strand with thin walls covered by a single layer of epithelial-like cells of hobnail pattern. Another common feature seen is a meshwork pattern with round hyaline globules that reacts to a-fetoprotein (AFP) in addition to other multiple pattern such as glandular, alveolar, hepatoid and myxomatous [10].

Teratomas are considered to arise from a single germ cell following the first meiotic division, with each of the three germ cell layers represented and consisting of both mature and immature elements. The histologic grade of immature teratomas is based on the presence of neuroepithelial components, the quantity of the neuroepithelial component and the degree of immaturity. Mature teratomas on the other hand are either cystic, constituting 99% or solid accounting for the remaining 1%. Solid mature teratoma usually constitutes tissues from all three cell layers with a well-differentiated glial component. The benign cystic teratoma that shows squamous epithelial involvement, and mesodermal and endodermal differentiation is usually benign, only a minute percentage undergo malignant progression to form squamous cell carcinoma [10, 15].

Mixed germ cell tumours include gonadoblastoma which is usually benign but sometimes associated with endodermal sinus tumour, embryonal carcinoma, choriocarcinoma or dysgerminoma.

4. Endometrioid ovarian cancer

Endometrioid ovarian carcinoma (EOVC) is an uncommon subtype of epithelial ovarian carcinoma (EOC) that constitute approximately 10% of all ovarian carcinomas. EOVC tends to present at a younger age and earlier stage, are associated with endometriosis, frequent *CTNNB1* and *PTEN* mutations and a higher frequency of microsatellite instability. Also, both the molecular and histologic makeup of EOVC is analogous to that of endometrioid endometrial carcinoma [6, 16].

5. High-grade serous ovarian carcinoma

5.1 Origin and epidemiology of high-grade serous ovarian cancer

EOC genomic predisposition is now recognized in about 15% of affected women, where Breast cancer susceptibility genes *BRCA1* and *BRCA2* were identified as the main causative agents of hereditary EOC. Different forms of mutations in these genes and other double-strand DNA break repair genes are mainly associated with susceptibility to HGSOC [1].

High-grade serous ovarian cancer (HGSOC) is the most common form of EOC, accounting for about 75% of all EOC (**Figure 1**). It has been found to originate from the fallopian tube epithelium due to its link with IGF-1R/AKT pathway, which is activated by follicular fluid [17]. However, the molecular basis of how it is transferred to the ovaries is yet to be understood. A recent study revealed that follicular fluid plays a vital role in events leading to the development and intraperitoneal metastasis of HGCOS, by supporting migration, proliferation, invasion, anchorage, adhesion and anoikis insensitivity [18].

5.2 Hereditary susceptibility

A study revealed that 15–20% of HGSOC patients have germline *BRCA1* and/or *BRCA2* mutations, which necessitates conducting germline testing on first-degree

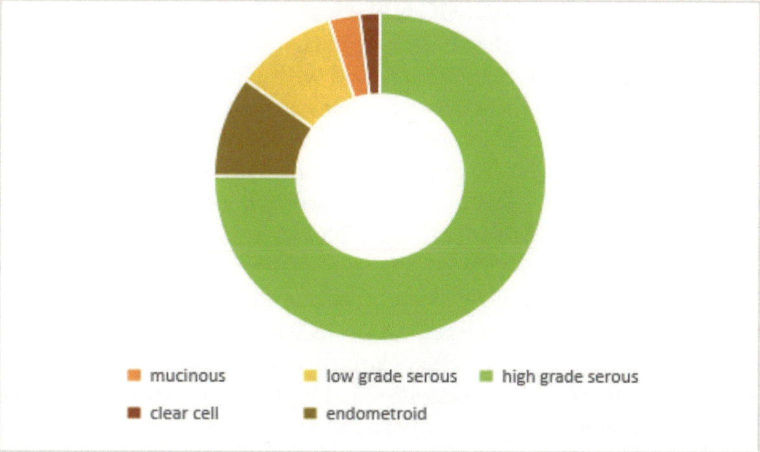

Figure 1.
Histologic distribution of ovarian cancer.

relatives to identify carriers [19]. Furthermore, it has been found that by the age of 80, the cumulative risk of EOC is about 44% and 17% in *BRCA1* and *BRCA2* mutation carriers respectively [20]. Therefore, such carriers are recommended to have a prophylactic risk-reduction surgery after childbearing, when the risk begins to increase. Apart from the above-mentioned genes, other genes with moderate penetrance include *RAD51C, RAD51D,* and *BR1P1*, which cumulatively are responsible for about 5% of EOC. Thus, genetic testing for HGSOC includes *BRCA1, BRCA2, RAD51C, RAD51D, BR1P1* and in the nearest future *TP53* detection in blood and uterine lavage [1, 21].

5.3 Pathology/molecular abnormality

The growth pattern of HGSOC is diverse, encompassing glandular, solid, large papillae with high mitotic rate and frequent necrosis [21]. HGSOC is characterized by recurrent mutations in *RB1, CDK12, BRCA1, BRCA2, NF1 and TP53*, and also frequent DNA losses and gains. This makes it chromosomally unstable with the potential of developing acquired chemoresistance [22, 23]. Thus, the homozygous and heterozygous loss is an important mechanism in tumour suppressor genes inactivation [1]. Also, studies have shown that homologous recombination is defective in almost half of HGSOC, and this deficiency is a key determinant of platinum sensitivity and treatment with Poly ADP-ribose polymerase inhibitors (PARPi) [22, 24]. HGSOC can be molecularly stratified into four different prognostic subtypes namely: mesenchymal-C1, immune-C2, differentiated-C4, and proliferative-C5, and into seven copy-number signatures [22, 25–27].

6. Recurrent clear cell ovarian carcinoma

Clear cell ovarian cancers (CCOC) are a subtype of EOC with very distinct biology to HGSOC. They exhibit a very poor prognosis and a low response to platinum-based chemotherapy. This subtype is molecularly heterogeneous for point mutations, gene copy number, and alterations in the *PI3K/AKT/mTOR* pathway. Thus, these could affect response to targeted therapy [28, 29]. Histologically, patients with CCOC must be correctly diagnosed because HGSOC with clear cell features can easily be misdiagnosed as CCOC [30]. This might also result in the decreased or failed response to treatment in such CCOC patients misdiagnosed with HGSOC.

A tumour profiling study to identify potential druggable targets in CCOC was carried out by employing protein expression by immunohistochemistry (IHC), next-generation sequencing (NGS) and gene amplification by fluorescent in situ hybridization (FISH). On the basis of IHC, this study revealed an 80.8% *RRM1* loss, 79.6% *ERCC1* loss, 56.4% *MGMT* loss, 50.8% *TS* loss and a 62.6% *TOP2A* overexpression [31]. The NGS identified 50.5%, 18.1%, and 12.4% mutations in *PIK3CA, TP53, and KRAS* respectively. Of which *TP53* mutations were observed on exons 4 to 8, while most *PIK3CA* mutations occurred on exons 9 and 20. For FISH analyses, *HER2* was amplified in 9.3% of pure and 3.8% of mixed CCOC samples, while *cMET*, was amplified in 3.2% of pure CCOC and none was amplified in mixed CCOC. Mutations in *ATM* and *APC* were also observed only in pure CCOC tumours [31].

Even though CCOCs are mostly chemoresistant, few patients do respond to platinum chemotherapy. Different mechanisms of CCOC chemoresistance have been reported including increased drug detoxification, increased DNA repair, decreased drug detoxification, abnormal growth factor signalling and cell cycle control. Loss of ARID 1A expression and alterations in the *PI3K/AKT/mTOR* pathway may also contribute to the chemoresistance in CCOC [32–34]. The *PI3K/AKT/mTOR* is a key mediator of oncogenic signalling, which may be overactive due to *PTEN* loss. The *PI3K* pathway is a complex signalling network that coordinates signals from other membrane receptors such as *MET* [35].

It is important to note that the signalling pathway of the receptor tyrosine kinase *MET* and its ligand hepatocyte growth factor (HGF) is crucial for cell motility, growth and survival, and is functionally linked to the *VEGF* signalling pathway [31]. Therefore, research into the kinase inhibitor agents that target *MET*, *VEGF* receptor 2 and other tyrosine kinases are urgently needed.

7. *TP53*: function and the consequence of its mutations in ovarian cancers

The *TP53* gene is a tumour suppressor gene located on the short arm of chromosome 17 and contains 11 exons that encode for 53 kDa phosphoprotein (*TP53* protein), a transcription factor of genes responsible for cell cycle arrest and apoptosis. It is a nuclear transcriptional factor that upon binding to the nucleic acid component of the cell, it facilitates the regulation of several cellular processes through the control of several expression genes to maintain overall genome integrity and homeostasis [36].

Following deoxyribonucleic acid (DNA) damage, the *TP53* gene initiates the activation of DNA repair proteins by arresting cell growth by holding the cell cycle at the G1/S transitioning phase. This allows DNA repairs and the initiation of apoptosis on cells with irreparable DNA damage [37]. The activation of *TP53* function has been associated with numerous carcinogenesis-inducing stimuli which induce DNA damage such as Gamma or UV irradiation, nucleolar or ribosomal stress, hypoxia, inappropriate activation of proto-oncogenes and mitogenic signalling among others [38–40]. Once initiated, the *TP53* through the promotion of expression of the necessary genes responsible for cellular damage regulatory activities, where appropriate initiates cell cycle arrest, cellular senescence and differentiation, and cell death [41, 42]. For example, upon DNA damage, the *TP53* protein binds to the damaged DNA and stimulates another cell cycle regulatory gene (CDKN1A) to produce *p21* protein which interacts and forms a complex with cyclin-dependent kinase 2 (*CDK2),* a cell division-stimulating protein [43]. The formed *CDKN1A-CDK2* complex arrests the affected cell and stopped its progression past the G1- phase of the cell cycle and induces cellular senescence [41, 42, 44]. This *TP53*-dependent blocking of cellular proliferation contributes to the prevention of cell transformation and tumour progression by triggering programmed cell death either by apoptosis or ferroptosis [36, 45]. However, an aberration in the *TP53* gene might result in the cessation of its cell cycle regulation and promotes carcinogenesis [46]. Therefore, these anti-tumour functions of *TP53* on DNA-damaged cells could be utilized for the development of anticancer drugs and appropriate management strategies.

TP53 is one of the most frequently mutated genes in human cancer with more than 50% of human cancer types associated with its mutations [47]. This is because of its essential role in DNA damage-induced cellular regulation and tumour suppression. There are over 36,000 *TP53* mutations identified of which approximately 80% of them are missense mutations with amino acid substitution [47]. According to IARC *TP53* Database, 6.5% of the identified *TP53* mutations have been reported to be associated with ovarian cancer of which approximately 70% of them are of the missense mutation subtypes while others include point and null mutations. Many of the missense mutations occurred at specific residues in the DNA binding domain which suggests a feature of selectivity peculiar to these mutants (http://www-TP53.iarc.fr/).

The mechanism underlying the development and progression of ovarian cancers as it relates to *TP53* mutation has been extensively studied. However, it is not well understood and researchers have suggested possible ways of its action. For example, one mechanism explored by researchers is the gain of function property. Mutant *TP53* acquires a "gain of function" property that favours ovarian cancer progressive activities that may manifest as acquired resistance to chemotherapy, enhanced invasiveness which positively increased metastatic capabilities and down-regulation of certain metabolic pathways among others [48]. The gain of function property of the mutant *TP53* can be observed in the abrogation of function upon interaction with its family members such as *p63* and *p73*. They both can form complexes with the Wild-type *TP53* and serve the tumour suppressor functions in cells [49]. However, mutant *TP53* with a gain of function property has been reported to form a complex with phosphorylated *p63* which prevents the Wild-type *p63* natural function of tumour suppression, and at the same time induces the activation of certain oncogenic genes such as Cyclin G2 and Dicer [50–52]. Similarly, a study reported that mutant *TP53* directly binds to Wild-type *p73* and as a result, it prevents the inactivation of PDGFβ- the natural function of the *p73*- which subsequently favours invasiveness and metastasis [53]. Another possible mechanism of mutant *TP53*-induced ovarian carcinogenesis may be associated with protein aggregation [54]. This is because the *TP53* mutants especially of the missense subtype category have been reported to induce structural changes which potentially expose adhesion molecules that can co-aggregate with the Wild-type *TP53* or any of its family members causing trans- or cis-DN effects on the Wild-types *TP53* and its analogues [54–56]. This can explain the reason certain ovarian cancers present with an aggregation phenotype and as such, they are considered aggregation-associated diseases by some scholars. In light of the aforementioned possible mechanisms by which mutant *TP53* aid in the development and progression of ovarian cancer, and the near 100% prevalence of this mutation in the high-grade serous ovarian cancer- the most prevalent type of ovarian cancer- type, it can be deduced that the *TP53* mutation in ovarian cancers presents with an opportunity worthy of exploring in therapeutic interventions and inhibition studies.

8. Conclusion

With Ovarian cancer being the 8th most common cancer among women globally, and one of the most complex diseases with multiple types each having distinct aetiology, risk factors and distinct response to treatment, tremendous progress has been so far recorded in understanding the molecular profiles of each type as well as the role played by *TP53* mutation in the development and progression of ovarian cancers. Also, understanding epidemiology, histopathology, and hereditary susceptibility are of equal importance.

Therefore, further molecular and biochemical studies that will explain detailed mechanisms underlying the role of the mutant *TP53* in ovarian cancer development and progression, especially the high-grade serous ovarian carcinoma are recommended. More so, further studies on the *TP53* mutation types will favour the development of the right therapeutic interventions for ovarian cancers.

Conflict of interest

The authors declare that they have no competing interests.

Author details

Imam Malik Kabir[1*] and Abdulaziz Tahir Idris[1,2]

1 Histopathology Unit, Department of Medical Laboratory Science, Bayero University, Kano, Nigeria

2 University of Chester, Chester, Cheshire, United Kingdom

*Address all correspondence to: imammkabir@yahoo.com

References

[1] Lheureux S, Charlie G, Vergote I, Oza AM. Epithelial ovarian cancer. Lancet. 2019;**393**:1240-1253

[2] Bast RC, Hennessy B, Mills GB. The biology of ovarian cancer: New opportunities for translation. Nature Reviews. Cancer. 2009;**9**(6):415. DOI: 10.1038/nrc2644

[3] Reid BM, Permuth JB, Sellers TA. Epidemiology of ovarian cancer: A review. Cancer Biology & Medicine. 2017;**14**:9-32. DOI: 10.20892/j.issn.2095-3941.2016.0084

[4] Vang R, Shih IM, Kurman RJ. Fallopian tube precursors of ovarian low- and high-grade serous neoplasms. Histopathology. 2013;**62**:44-58

[5] Ksiaz˙ek K. Molecular biology of ovarian cancer: From mechanisms of intraperitoneal metastasis to therapeutic opportunities. Cancers. 2021;**13**:1661. DOI: 10.3390/cancers13071661

[6] Cybulska P, Paula ADC, Tseng J, Leitao MM Jr, Bashashati A, Huntsman DG, et al. Molecular profiling and molecular classification of endometrioid ovarian carcinomas. Gynecologic Oncology. 2019;**154**(3):516-523. DOI: 10.1016/j.ygyno.2019.07.012

[7] Shih IM, Kurman RJ. Ovarian tumorigenesis—A proposedmodel based onmorphological and molecular genetic analysis. The American Journal of Pathology. 2004;**164**:1511-1518

[8] Banerjee S, Kaye SB. New strategies in the treatment of ovarian cancer: Current clinical perspectives and future potential. Clinical Cancer Research. 2013;**19**:961-968

[9] Wang YK, Bashashati A, Anglesio MS, Cochrane DR, Grewal DS, Ha G, et al. Genomic consequences of aberrant DNA repair mechanisms stratify ovarian cancer histotypes. Nature Genetics. 2017;**49**:856-865

[10] Gore H. Histopathology of ovarian cancer. Seminars in Surgical Oncology. 1994;**10**:255-260

[11] Kurman RJ, Trimble CL. The behavior of serous tumors of low malignant potential: Are they ever malignant? International Journal of Gynecological Pathology. 1993;**12**:120-127

[12] Montag AG, Jenison EL, Griffiths CT, Welch WR, Lavin PT, Knapp RC. Ovarian clear cell carcinoma. A clinicopathologic analysis of 44 cases. International Journal of Gynecological Pathology. 1989;**8**(2):85-96

[13] Imachi M, Tsukamoto N, Shimamoto T, Hirakawa T, Vehira K, Nakano H. Clear cell carcinoma of the ovary: A clinicopathologic analysis of 34 cases. International Journal of Gynecological Cancer. 1991;**1**:113-119

[14] Bell DA, Scully RE. Benign and borderline clear cell adenofibroma of the ovary. Cancer. 1985;**56**:2922-2931

[15] Talerman A. Germ cell tumors of the ovary. In: Kurman RJ, editor. Blaustein's Pathology of the Female Genital Tract. 3rd ed. New York: Springer-Verlag; 1987. pp. 659-721

[16] Pierson WE, Peters PN, Chang MT, Chen L, Quigley DA, Ashworth A, et al. An integrated molecular profile of endometrioid ovarian cancer. Gynecologic Oncology. 2020;**157**:55-61

[17] Ducie J, Dao F, Considine M, Olvera N, Shaw PA, Kurman RJ, et al. Molecular analysis of high-grade serous ovarian carcinoma with and without associated serous tubal intra-epithelial carcinoma. Nature Communications. 2017;**8**:990

[18] Hsu CF, Chen PC, Seenan V, Ding DC, Chu TY. Ovulatory follicular fluid facilitates the full transformation process for the development of high-grade serous carcinoma. Cancers. 2021;**13**:468

[19] Alsop K, Fereday S, Meldrum C, et al. BRCA mutation frequency and patterns of treatment response in BRCA mutation-positive women with ovarian cancer: A report from the Australian ovarian cancer study group. Journal of Clinical Oncology. 2012;**30**:2654-2663

[20] Kuchenbaecker KB, Hopper JL, Barnes DR, et al. Risks of breast, ovarian, and contralateral breast cancer for BRCA1 and BRCA2 mutation carriers. JAMA. 2017;**317**:2402-2416

[21] Widschwendter M, Zikan M, Wahl B, et al. The potential of circulating tumor DNA methylation analysis for the early detection and management of ovarian cancer. Genome Medicine. 2017;**9**:116

[22] The Cancer Genome Atlas Research Network. Integrated genomic analyses of ovarian carcinoma. Nature. 2011;**474**:609-615

[23] Bowtell DD, Böhm S, Ahmed AA, et al. Rethinking ovarian cancer II: Reducing mortality from high-grade serous ovarian cancer. Nature Reviews. Cancer. 2015;**15**:668-679

[24] Scott CL, Swisher EM, Kaufmann SH. Poly (ADP-ribose) polymerase inhibitors: Recent advances and future development. Journal of Clinical Oncology. 2015;**33**:1397-1406

[25] Tothill RW, Tinker AV, George J, et al. And the Australian ovarian cancer study group. Novel molecular subtypes of serous and endometrioid ovarian cancer linked to clinical outcome. Clinical Cancer Research. 2008;**14**:5198-5208

[26] Konecny GE, Wang C, Hamidi H, et al. Prognostic and therapeutic relevance of molecular subtypes in high-grade serous ovarian cancer. Journal of the National Cancer Institute. 2014;**106**:dju249

[27] Macintyre G, Goranova T, De Silva D, et al. Copy-number signatures and mutational processes in ovarian carcinoma. Nature Genetics. 2018;**50**:1262-1270

[28] Tan DS, Miller RE, Kaye SB. New perspectives on molecular targeted therapy in ovarian clear cell carcinoma. British Journal of Cancer. 2013;**108**:1553-1559

[29] Tan DS, Iravani M, McCluggage WG, et al. Genomic analysis reveals the molecular heterogeneity of ovarian clear cell carcinomas. Clinical Cancer Research. 2011;**17**:1521-1534

[30] Han G, Gilks CB, Leung S, et al. Mixed ovarian epithelial carcinomas with clear cell and serous components are variants of high-grade serous carcinoma: An interobserver correlative and immunohistochemical study of 32 cases. The American Journal of Surgical Pathology. 2008;**32**:955-964

[31] Friedlander ML, Russell K, Millis S, Gatalica Z, Bender R, Voss A. Molecular profiling of clear cell ovarian CancersIdentifying potential treatment targets for clinical trials. International

Journal of Gynecologic Cancer. 2016;**26**(4):648-654

[32] Burris HA. Overcoming acquired resistance to anticancer therapy: Focus on the *PI3K/AKT/mTOR* pathway. Cancer Chemotherapy and Pharmacology. 2013;**71**:829-842

[33] Itamochi H, Kigawa J, Terakawa N. Mechanisms of chemoresistance and poor prognosis in ovarian clear cell carcinoma. Cancer Science. 2008;**99**:653-658

[34] Katagiri A, Nakayama K, Rahman MT, et al. Loss of ARID1A expression is related to shorter progression-free survival and chemoresistance in ovarian clear cell carcinoma. Modern Pathology. 2012;**25**:282-288

[35] Takano M, Kouta H, Ikeda Y, et al. Combination chemotherapy with temsirolimus and trabectedin for recurrent clear cell carcinoma of the ovary: A phase II single arm clinical trial. Journal of Clinical Oncology. 2014;**32**(15):5517

[36] Hernández Borrero LJ, El-Deiry WS. Tumor suppressor *TP53*: Biology, signaling pathways, and therapeutic targeting. Biochimica et Biophysica Acta (BBA)—Reviews on. Cancer. 2021;**1876**(1):188556. DOI: 10.1016/j.bbcan.2021.188556

[37] Brosh R, Rotter V. When mutants gain new powers: News from the mutant *TP53* field. Nature Reviews Cancer. 2009;**9**(10):701-713. DOI: 10.1038/nrc2693

[38] Dai C, Gu W. *TP53* post-translational modification: Deregulated in tumorigenesis. Trends in Molecular Medicine. 2010;**16**(11):528-536. DOI: 10.1016/j.molmed.2010.09.002

[39] James A, Wang Y, Raje H, Rosby R, DiMario P. Nucleolar stress with and without *TP53*. Nucleus. 2014;**5**(5):402-426. DOI: 10.4161/nucl.32235

[40] Zhou X, Liao JM, Liao WJ, Lu H. Scission of the *TP53*-MDM2 loop by ribosomal proteins. Genes & Cancer. 2012;**3**(3-4):298-310. DOI: 10.1177/1947601912455200

[41] Chen J. The cell-cycle arrest and apoptotic functions of *TP53* in tumor initiation and progression. Cold Spring Harbor Perspectives in Medicine. 2016;**6**(3):a026104. DOI: 10.1101/cshperspect.a026104

[42] Rufini A, Tucci P, Celardo I, Melino G. Senescence and aging: The critical roles of *TP53*. Oncogene. 2013;**32**(43):5129-5143. DOI: 10.1038/onc.2012.640

[43] Lacroix M, Riscal R, Arena G, Linares LK, le Cam L. Metabolic functions of the tumor suppressor *TP53*: Implications in normal physiology, metabolic disorders, and cancer. Molecular Metabolism. 2020;**33**:2-22. DOI: 10.1016/j.molmet.2019.10.002

[44] Keshava C, Frye BL, Wolff MS, McCanlies EC, Weston A. Waf-1 (*p21*) and *TP53* polymorphisms in breast cancer. Cancer Epidemiology, Biomarkers & Prevention. 2002;**11**(1):127-130

[45] Jiang L, Kon N, Li T, Wang SJ, Su T, Hibshoosh H, et al. Ferroptosis as a *TP53*-mediated activity during tumour suppression. Nature. 2015;**520**(7545):57-62. DOI: 10.1038/nature14344

[46] Nobili S, Bruno L, Landini I, Napoli C, Bechi P, Tonelli F, et al. Genomic and genetic alterations influence the progression of gastric cancer. World Journal of

Gastroenterology. 2011;**17**(3):290-299. DOI: 10.3748/wjg.v17.i3.290

[47] Zhang Y, Cao L, Nguyen D, Lu H. *TP53* mutations in epithelial ovarian cancer. Translational Cancer Research. 2016;**5**(6):650-663. DOI: 10.21037/tcr.2016.08.40

[48] Haupt Y, Maya R, Kazaz A, Oren M. Mdm2 promotes the rapid degradation of *TP53*. Nature. 1997;**387**(6630):296-299. DOI: 10.1038/387296a0

[49] Freed-Pastor WA, Prives C. Mutant *TP53*: One name, many proteins. Genes & Development. 2012;**26**(12):1268-1286. DOI: 10.1101/gad.190678.112

[50] Adorno M, Cordenonsi M, Montagner M, Dupont S, Wong C, Hann B, et al. A mutant-*TP53*/Smad complex opposes *p63* to empower TGFβ-induced metastasis. Cell. 2000;**137**(1):87-98. DOI: 10.1016/j.cell.2009.01.039

[51] Girardini JE, Napoli M, Piazza S, Rustighi A, Marotta C, Radaelli E, et al. A Pin1/mutant *TP53* Axis promotes aggressiveness in breast cancer. Cancer Cell. 2011;**20**(1):79-91. DOI: 10.1016/j.ccr.2011.06.004

[52] Su X, Chakravarti D, Cho MS, Liu L, Gi YJ, Lin YL, et al. TA*p63* suppresses metastasis through coordinate regulation of dicer and miRNAs. Nature. 2010;**467**(7318):986-990. DOI: 10.1038/nature09459

[53] Weissmueller S, Manchado E, Saborowski M, Morris JP, Wagenblast E, Davis CA, et al. Mutant *TP53* drives pancreatic cancer metastasis through cell-autonomous PDGF receptor β signaling. Cell. 2014;**157**(2):382-394. DOI: 10.1016/j.cell.2014.01.066

[54] Xu J, Reumers J, Couceiro JR, de Smet F, Gallardo R, Rudyak S, et al. Gain of function of mutant *TP53* by coaggregation with multiple tumor suppressors. Nature Chemical Biology. 2011;**7**(5):285-295. DOI: 10.1038/nchembio.546

[55] Rangel LP, Costa DC, Vieira TC, Silva JL. The aggregation of mutant *TP53* produces prion-like properties in cancer. Prion. 2014;**8**(1):75-84. DOI: 10.4161/pri.27776

[56] Silva JL, Rangel LP, Costa DCF, Cordeiro Y, de Moura Gallo CV. Expanding the prion concept to cancer biology: Dominant-negative effect of aggregates of mutant *TP53* tumour suppressor. Bioscience Reports. 2013;**33**(4):e00054. DOI: 10.1042/BSR20130065

Chapter 2

Recent Advances in Classification and Histopathological Diagnosis of Ovarian Epithelial Malignant Tumours

Gabriela-Monica Stanc, Efthymia Souka and Christos Valavanis

Abstract

Ovarian tumours are a heterogeneous group of neoplasms classified based on histopathologic type and grade of differentiation. They comprise a broad range of tumours from benign and borderline to malignant histotypes characterised by different histopathological, immunophenotypic and molecular features. The purpose of this chapter is to present an overview of the recent advances in the ovarian epithelial malignant tumours classification along with the histopathological, immunophenotypic and molecular diagnostic criteria highlighting areas of terminology discrepancies or changes and diagnostic challenges. These changes provide a better understanding of the ovarian tumours nature and lead to a more efficient therapeutic management of these pathological entities.

Keywords: ovarian cancer, histopathology, immunophenotype, molecular pathology

1. Introduction

Ovarian cancer is the most lethal malignancy of gynaecological cancer representing 23% of gynaecological neoplasms and the 5th most common leading cause of death in women. Most ovarian malignant neoplasms are diagnosed at an advanced stage with high recurrence rates and an overall 5-year survival rate of around 50% [1–3].

Ovarian tumours originate from ovarian or fallopian tube tissue and are divided into epithelial tumours (benign, border-line and malignant), germ cell tumours, sex cord-stromal tumours and mesenchymal tumours [4].

In this chapter, we will focus on the epithelial ovarian malignant tumours and will present an overview of the recent advances in the ovarian tumours classification along with their histopathological, immunophenotypic and molecular features.

Epithelial ovarian malignant tumours comprise a heterogeneous neoplastic disease with distinct histomorphologic features, pathogenesis, precursor lesions, immunophenotypic and molecular profiles, different biological behaviour and clinical outcomes [4]. According to the recent 2020 WHO classification based on histomorphology, immunophenotypic features and molecular alterations, epithelial ovarian malignant tumours are classified into five main types with different incidences: high-grade serous carcinoma (HGSC—70%), low-grade serous carcinoma (LGSC—5%), endometrioid (EC—10%), mucinous (MC—3%) and clear cell carcinomas (CCC—10%) [3–6].

Rare histopathologic entities are seromucinous carcinoma, malignant Brenner tumour, mesonephric-like carcinoma, undifferentiated and dedifferentiated carcinomas, carcinosarcoma and mixed cell carcinoma [5]. Seromucinous carcinoma as a distinct entity, characterised by serous and endocervical-type mucinous epithelium with foci of clear cells and areas of endometrioid and squamous differentiation, has been removed from the recent 2020 WHO classification. It is now considered a subtype of endometrioid carcinoma based on immunohistochemical and molecular studies [5].

Traditional concepts of ovarian carcinogenesis assumed that ovarian cancer pathogenesis is due to Müllerian or non-Müllerian metaplasia of ovarian surface epithelium leading progressively to malignant transformation [7] or due to malignant transformation of endometriosis lesions and/or inclusion cysts [8]. Recent pathological observations and molecular studies have revealed that the majority of the high-grade serous carcinomas arise from a precursor dysplastic lesion in the fimbria of fallopian tubes, designated as STIC (Serous Tubal Intraepithelial Carcinoma), whereas low-grade serous carcinomas arise within the ovarian parenchyma from benign or borderline serous tumours [9–11]. In addition, the presence of genomic alterations in the *BRCA1* and *BRCA2* tumour suppressor genes and gene mutations in *p53, p16, CCNE1, BRD4* and *RSF1,* and centrosome copy number abnormalities, in STIC and high-grade serous carcinoma, suggest a clonal histogenetic relationship between this precursor lesion and HGSC [12–15]. A clonal histogenetic relationship has also been observed among endometriosis, precursor ovarian surface epithelium lesions and endometrioid and clear cell carcinomas based on mutations found in *ARID1A, PIK3CA, KRAS* and *MET* genes among these pathologic entities [16–18].

It is now well established that ovarian carcinogenesis is based on a dualistic model of pathogenesis that divides ovarian epithelial malignant tumours into two main categories, designated as type I and type II ovarian tumours [7].

Type I ovarian epithelial tumours arise from precursor lesions in the ovary such as cystadenoma or adenofibroma. These lesions can undergo malignant transformation through atypical proliferation or transformation to borderline tumours and eventually into invasive ovarian neoplasms. Type I ovarian epithelial tumours include low-grade serous carcinoma, endometrioid carcinoma, mucinous carcinoma, clear cell carcinoma and malignant Brenner tumour. They have a relatively indolent clinical course and are characterised by genomic stability, distinctive molecular profile for each histotype and low incidence of p53 mutations (10–13%), except of mucinous carcinoma, which displays high incidence of p53 mutations (64%) [19, 20].

Type II ovarian epithelial tumours arise from distal fallopian tube fimbria epithelium through dysplastic lesions (STIC) and finally towards invasive carcinomas. They show aggressive biological behaviour and comprise high-grade serous carcinoma, carcinosarcoma and dedifferentiated and undifferentiated carcinomas [6, 21]. They are characterised by genomic instability, high incidence of p53 mutations and abnormal function of tumour suppressor genes *BRCA1* and *BRCA2* due to mutations or gene promoter hypermethylation [19, 20].

In the following sections, we are going to present the morphologic, immunophenotypic and molecular alterations that can be found in the five main histotypes of ovarian epithelial malignant tumours and the putative implications that may have in the clinical outcomes and targeted therapeutic interventions.

2. High-grade serous ovarian carcinomas (HGSCs)

High-grade serous carcinomas (HGSCs) account for 70% of ovarian carcinomas and represent the most aggressive and chemoresistant epithelial ovarian neoplasms. Most patients are postmenopausal women and admitted to the hospital at advanced clinical stage (80%) with extra-ovarian metastasis and thus with a high incidence of mortality around 70–80% globally [22].

Common predisposition factors are infertility, menopausal hormonal therapy and the hereditary breast and ovarian cancer (HBOC) syndrome characterised mostly by germline *BRCA1/2* genomic alterations [23] and less frequently (2%) by germline genomic alterations in other homologous recombination repair (HRR) genes such as *ATM, BRIP1, RAD51C* and *RAD51D* [24, 25].

2.1 Pathology of ovarian high-grade serous carcinomas

These tumours are large, exophytic and usually bilateral with solid and papillary growth patterns and fluid-containing cysts. Necrosis is not uncommon and extraovarian affected sites can be observed. Occasionally a small tumour nodule can be found at the distal part of the fallopian tube fimbria.

Microscopically, HGSCs are heterogeneous tumours displaying solid, papillary, glandular and/or cribriform architectural patterns, sometimes with slit-like spaces. Recently, two histotypes have been observed, the classic type and the SET type (solid pseudoendometrioid and transitional variant) [5]. Classic type HGSCs exhibit papillary, micropapillary and solid growth patterns. The neoplastic cells demonstrate large pleomorphic nuclei with prominent nucleoli, high mitotic activity (>5 mitoses/mm^2) including atypical mitoses and presence of multinucleated cells. SET type HGSCs are characterised by solid sheets of neoplastic cells mimicking endometrioid and/or transitional cell carcinomas, sometimes with bizarre cytologic features. Occasionally a micropapillary pattern can be seen and areas with geographical necrosis can be also found. These tumours are associated with a high number of tumour infiltrating lymphocytes (TILs) [5, 26]. SET pattern is more commonly correlated with germline and/or somatic *BRCA1/2* mutations [26] and is more sensitive to chemotherapy and PARP inhibitors.

Based on *BRCA* mutation status, histomorphological patterns (classic vs. SET), STIC presence and clinical outcome, two categories of HGSC can be identified: (1) BRCA-mutated tumours exhibiting SET morphology, absence of STIC lesions, more common in young patients, more chemosensitive and responsive to PARP inhibitors with favourable prognosis and (2) tumours without *BRCA* genomic alterations displaying classic morphology, presence of STIC lesions, more common in old aged patients and less responsive to chemotherapy with unfavourable clinical outcome [26, 27].

The WHO 2020 classification introduces specific criteria for site assignment of HGSCs origin (fallopian tube, ovary, tubo-ovarian or peritoneal) **Table 1** [5]. According to these criteria, 80% of the cases are of tubal origin, whereas peritoneal

Primary site	Criteria for diagnosis
Fallopian tube	Presence of STIC or Presence of invasive fallopian tube HGSC or Part or entire fallopian tube length inseparable from tubo-ovarian tumor
Ovary	Both fallopian tubes separable from ovarian tumor and No STIC or invasive HGSC in either fallopian tube examined by SEE-FM (sectioning and extensively examining the tubal fimbria)
Tubo-ovarian	Fallopian tubes and ovaries not available for full examination and Pathological findings consistent with extrauterine HGSC
Peritoneal	Both tubes and both ovaries fully examined and No gross or microscopic evidence of STIC or HGSC in tubes or ovaries

Table 1.
Criteria for assigning primary site in high grade serous carcinomas.

origin should be considered only after careful exclusion of STIC and absence of ovarian involvement.

2.2 Immunophenotypic features of ovarian high-grade serous carcinomas

Immunohistochemical analysis should be performed in order to distinguish ovarian high-grade serous carcinoma from mesothelioma or other poorly differentiated carcinomas in cases of peritoneal carcinomatosis. It can also be useful in small biopsies and in post-therapy specimens.

Both classical and SET HGSC histotypes show positive immunoreactivity against CK7, p16, PAX8, WT1, ER (oestrogen receptor) and PgR (progesterone receptor), and this panel of antibodies is enough to establish an ovarian serous carcinoma diagnosis [5]. In addition, 30–50% of HGSCs can exhibit three different aberrant expression patterns for p53, strong, diffuse nuclear overexpression in >80% of cells associated with TP53 missense mutation, no expression implying p53 loss of function and diffuse cytoplasmic expression with weak nuclear intensity similar to wild-type immunoreactivity correlated with loss of function mutations disrupting the nuclear localization signal domain [28, 29]. Strong positive p53 immunoreactivity can also help to identify foci of intraepithelial carcinoma on the ovarian surface or in the fallopian tube epithelium (STIC). HGSCs also exhibit cytoplasmic and/or nuclear p16 expression along with a high Ki-67 (MIB-1) cell proliferation index (>75%) [30].

Ovarian HGSCs can be differentiated from mesotheliomas using a panel of various antibodies such as PAX8, Ber-EP4, MOC-31, ER (positive expression in ovarian serous carcinomas) and Calretinin, CK5/6 (both positive in mesotheliomas) [31].

Diagnostic problem can arise between HGSC of solid morphologic patterns and a poorly differentiated endometrioid carcinoma. In such a case serous carcinoma displays diffuse strong staining for WT1, p53 and p16 [32, 33].

Serous carcinoma of the endometrium shows negative or focally weakly positive WT1 immunoreactivity but p53 positive, therefore, metastatic serous carcinoma with this immunophenotype should be considered endometrial than ovarian origin [33].

WT1 immunopositivity is also observed in serous borderline tumours and in sex cord-stromal tumours [34, 35]. On the other hand, serous borderline and benign tumours show negative immunoreactivity for p53 [29, 33].

2.3 Molecular pathology of ovarian high-grade serous carcinomas

Massive parallel sequencing studies have revealed that ovarian HGSCs are characterised by somatic *TP53* mutations more commonly in the DNA binding domain in high frequency (>95%) [36, 37]. They have also demonstrated genomic alterations in the homologous recombination repair (HRR) pathway leading to genomic instability and aneuploidy characterised by high copy number structural alterations (CNAs). CNAs can be recognised as oncogene amplifications such as *CCNE1* (20%), *MECOM, EMSY* and *MYC* and deletions/breaks of tumour suppressor genes such as *PTEN, RB1, RAD51B* and *NF1* [38, 39]. Additionally, recurrent mutations have been observed in a variety of genes such as *NF1* (4%–6%), *RB1* (2%–6%)and *PTEN* (<1%) along with structural alterations/deletions can result in genes inactivation in relatively high frequency such as 20%, 17% and 7%, respectively [38, 40]. Ovarian HGSCs display genomic alterations in *BRCA1/2* genes that are involved in the homologous recombination repair (HRR) pathway. Almost 15% of HGSCs have *BRCA1/2* germline mutations, 5% somatic mutations and 11% show *BRCA1* promoter epigenetic silencing through CpG islands hypermethylation [38, 41]. Mutational alterations have also been observed in other HRR-related genes resulting in an HRR deficient phenotype in 50% of the cases and leading to high genomic instability [42]. These HRR-related genes include Fanconi anaemia genes (*PALB2, FANCA, FANC1, FANCL, FANCC*), *RAD* family genes (*RAD50, RAD51, RAD51B, RAD51C, RAD54L*), MRN complex genes [*Mrc11-Rad50-Nbs1(Nibrin)*] and DNA damage response (DDR) genes (*ATM, ATR, CHEK1, CHEK2*) [42, 43]. Based on the HRR pathway status, HGSCs can be categorised into two morphologically distinct histotypes. *HRR- proficient tumours* demonstrate papillary, micropapillary and slit-like space architectural patterns with worse prognosis, while *HRR-deficient (HRD) tumours* show SET-like morphology (solid, endometrioid and transitional patterns) and improved progression-free survival due to beneficial responsiveness to platinum and poly ADP-ribose polymerase (PARP) inhibitors [26, 44]. HRR-proficient tumours are more likely to be resistant to these therapeutic interventions and are characterised by genomic alterations unrelated and mutually exclusive to *BRCA1/2* pathway, such as *CCNE1* gene amplification [45, 46].

According to NCCN guidelines HRD status should be tested in order to optimise the PARP inhibitor HGSCs treatment. Most of the HRD assays evaluate the status of germline or somatic HRR gene mutations and the presence of genomic instability by analysing the percentage of genomic loss of heterozygosity, telomeric allelic imbalance and genome-wide structural alterations (HRD mutation signatures) [47–49]. It should be noted that primary resistance to PARP inhibition can be observed in HGSCs with functional HRR, particularly in the presence of CCNE1 amplification. Additionally acquired resistance or decreased sensitivity to PARPi therapy can occur through HRR genes functional restoration by secondary mutations [50, 51]. In this setting, a functional assay can be used by evaluating the HRD status at RNA or protein levels [52, 53].

Other prognostic and treatment predictive biomarkers in HGSCs include tumour molecular subtyping based on transcriptional profiling that divides HGSCs into four categories (differentiated, immunoreactive, mesenchymal and proliferative), the former (differentiated and immunoreactive) with favourable biological behaviour and prognosis and the latter (mesenchymal and proliferative) with aggressive clinical course and worse prognosis [54–56]. In addition, promoter hypermethylation of *TAP1* gene in 6p21.3 chromosomal locus confers an unfavourable prognosis, while an increased count of CD8+ tumour infiltrating T lymphocytes is associated with favourable outcome [57–59]. Protein expression studies on PD-L1, LAG3 and potential use of immunotherapeutic modalities on ovarian HGSCs have demonstrated modest therapeutic results and controversial prognosis [60–62]. Other dysregulated pathways in HGSCs are the *PIK3CA/AKT* and *NOTCH* pathways which can be therapeutically targeted by using PIK3CA or AKT inhibitors [63, 64], whereas *HER2* overexpression/amplification (2–4% in HGSCs) has no significant impact on prognosis, albeit a finding that can be exploited for anti-HER2 targeted therapy [65, 66].

3. Low-grade serous ovarian carcinomas (LGSCs)

Low-grade serous carcinomas (LGSCs*)* are more common in younger women, with a median age of 43 years, have a better clinical course and prognosis than HGSCs and account for approximately 3–5% of epithelial ovarian tumours [67]. LSGCs originate from benign or borderline serous tumours and about 50% are associated with a borderline component. Progression of borderline serous tumour into low-grade serous carcinoma occurs in 6–7% of the cases and evolution to high grade serous carcinoma is rare. A more aggressive clinical course is associated with the presence of a borderline serous tumour component showing micropapillary histological pattern, microinvasions and bilateral ovarian presence [68].

3.1 Pathology of ovarian low-grade serous carcinomas

Macroscopically LGSCs are often bilateral and have a papillary appearance. Foci of calcification may be present. Microscopically, they display papillary, micropapillary, glandular, nested or inverted macropapillary architectural patterns- free-floating within unlined empty spaces, with a variety of invasion patterns. Neoplastic cells demonstrate low to moderate grade nuclear atypia with no pleomorphism (<3× size variation), distinct central nucleoli and relatively low mitotic activity (1–2 mitoses/mm^2). Necrosit areas are rare and psammoma bodies are frequent. LGSCs are differentiated from their serous borderline tumour component by the presence of stromal invasive foci measuring >5 mm or 10 mm^2 in size [5, 69].

3.2 Immunophenotypic features of ovarian low-grade serous carcinomas

LGSCs show positive immunoreactivity against CK7, PAX8, WT1, ER (oestrogen receptor) and PgR (progesterone receptor). Unlike HGSCs, they display patchy or negative expression for p16, low levels of Ki-67 proliferation index (less than 3%) and wild-type immunoreactivity for p53 [70].

3.3 Molecular pathology of ovarian low-grade serous carcinomas

LGSCs are characterised by genomic stability with low mutation rates, are not associated with *BRCA* germline genomic alterations and display low copy number genetic aberrations, like chromosomal loss of 1p36.33, 9p and homozygous deletions of the *CDKN2A/2B* locus in approximately 86% of LGSCs [71, 72].

The most common molecular alterations found in LGSCs have activated mutations of upstream regulators of MAPK signal transduction pathway like *KRAS* (25–54%), *BRAF* (8–33%), *NRAS* (8–26%) and *ERBB2* (5–6%) [4, 73]. *KRAS* and *BRAF* mutations are early events in LGSCs evolution and can be found in 85% of benign cystadenomas and serous borderline tumours [74]. *KRAS* mutations are associated with aggressive biological behaviour and unfavourable prognosis whereas *BRAF* mutations are found in early clinical stage [75, 76]. Other driver mutations involved in the pathogenetic mechanisms of LGSCs have been observed in *PIK3CA*, *FFAR1*, *MACF1* (11%), *USP9X* (11-27%), *ARID1A* (9%), *NF2* (4%), *DOT1L* (6%), *ASH1L* (4%) and *EIF1AX* (15%) [77]. *USPX9* and *EIF1AX* are downstream effectors of MAPK pathway and linked to the mTOR pathway. Therefore, mTOR inhibitors may be used for targeted therapies in chemoresistant recurrent tumours [78].

4. Ovarian endometrioid carcinomas (OECs)

Endometrioid ovarian carcinomas account for 10–15% of epithelial ovarian tumours are correlated with favourable prognosis and can be found in women ageing 30–80 years [79]. They arise mainly from endometriosis lesions and less frequently from benign or borderline endometrioid ovarian neoplasms, such as adenofibromas or endometrioid borderline tumours [80]. Atypical endometriosis is the precursor lesion for 40% of OECs. Risk factors for OECs are endometriosis lesions, Lynch syndrome, hereditary breast and ovarian cancer syndrome, late menopause and postmenopausal hormone therapy [80, 81].

4.1 Pathology of ovarian endometrioid carcinomas

Endometrioid carcinomas of the ovary present mainly as unilateral mass in the ovary and less frequently as bilateral (20%) [82]. They display a smooth external surface and a solid/cystic cut surface, sometimes with a residual endometriotic cyst at the periphery of the tumour [80]. Microscopically, these tumours show a variety of morphologic patterns such as glandular, cribriform, villoglandular or solid with characteristic back-to-back glands, areas of squamous differentiation and expansile rather than an infiltrative pattern of invasion [5]. Sometimes a destructive invasion pattern can be seen characterised by neoplastic cells infiltrating the stroma accompanied by a desmoplastic reaction. The neoplastic cells are tall columnar and focally mucinous with a mitotic activity of 5–10 mitoses per high power field [5, 82]. Histologic characteristics confirmatory of OECs are metaplastic features such as squamous, morular, hobnail or mucinous metaplasia, presence of endometriosis lesions, ovarian endometrioid adenofibroma or endometrioid borderline tumour, and presence of a synchronous uterine endometrioid carcinoma found in 15–20% of the cases [5]. Ovarian endometrioid carcinomas are divided according to the presence of solid growth pattern in grade 1 (less than 5% solid growth), grade 2 (5–50% solid growth) and grade 3 (more than 50% solid growth), excluding areas of squamous differentiation [5].

4.2 Immunophenotypic features of ovarian endometrioid carcinomas

OECs show diffuse immunopositivity for CK7, PAX8, ER and PgR [83]. Approximately 33% of OECs display membranous and/or cytoplasmic diffuse expression for vimentin [84]. Squamous morules of endometrioid tumours demonstrate strong CD10 cytoplasmic expression [85] and infrequently CDX2 immunopositive reaction [86]. Endometrioid ovarian carcinomas also exhibit β-catenin membranous and/or cytoplasmic expression. Nuclear β-catenin expression is correlated with *CTNNB1* genomic alterations and favourable prognosis [77]. Differential diagnosis between high-grade endometrioid carcinomas with solid architectural patterns and high-grade serous carcinomas can be made based on the intense diffuse immunopositivity of WT1, p53 and p16 in HGSCs, whereas ECs display patchy expression for p16, wild-type or mutation-type expression for p53 and loss of WT1 immunoreactivity [87].

4.3 Molecular pathology of ovarian endometrioid carcinomas

OECs are characterised mainly by mutations in *PIK3CA* (15–40%), *ARID1A* (30–35%), a component of the SW1/SNF chromatin remodelling complex, *KRAS* (10–30%) and *CTNNB1* (25–60%) involved in the WNT/β-catenin signal transduction pathway [88–90]. Borderline endometrioid ovarian tumours have *CTNNB1* mutations in 90% of the cases [77, 90]. Other less common genomic alterations are mutations in *PTEN* (20–30%) with frequent loss of heterozygosity (45–75%), *TP53* (10–25%) and *POLE* (3–10%) [91, 92]. Somatic or germline predisposition mutations in MMR genes (MLH1, MSH2, MSH6, PMS2) can be found in 10–20% of the cases, some of them associated with Lynch syndrome [93, 94]. *POLE*-mutated EOCs and MMR-deficient ovarian endometrioid tumours have favourable clinical outcomes [95, 96]. *CTNNB1*-mutated tumours show low genomic complexity and are correlated with low-grade tumours and good prognosis, unlike their uterine endometrioid counterparts, which demonstrate worse clinical outcomes [77, 97]. *TP53* mutated EOCs have high genomic complexity with poor prognosis [98]. Synchronous presence of endometrial and ovarian endometrioid carcinomas can be encountered in 25% of the cases demonstrating a putative clonal relationship with favourable prognosis [99, 100]. Ovarian seromucinous carcinomas (mixed serous and endocervical-type mucinous carcinomas) are considered by the current WHO classification a subtype of endometrioid ovarian carcinomas based on their morphological and molecular overlapping features [5, 101, 102]. Based on their molecular features, EOCs are divided into four molecular subcategories: 1. *hypermutated* with microsatellite instability due to MMR deficiency (10–20%), 2. *ultramutated* due to *POLE* exonuclease domain mutations (3–10%), 3. *TP53 mutated* (10–25%) and 4. with *no specific molecular signatures* (60–70%) [95, 103]. Hypermutated and ultramutated EOCs display high mutation burden, a molecular finding that might be exploited for immunotherapeutic interventions. The genomic aberrations identified in EOCs might be used as targets for therapeutic interventions, such as targeting mutated *ARID1A* with HDAC inhibitors or targeting dysregulated MAPK or PI3K pathways using MEK or PIK3AC inhibitors, respectively [104, 105].

5. Ovarian mucinous carcinomas (OMCs)

Primary ovarian mucinous tumours are relatively rare, approximately 10–15% of all ovarian tumours and most of them (80%) are benign or borderline mucinous tumours. Mucinous carcinomas in the ovary represent 3% of ovarian carcinomas with relatively high prevalence in women below 40 years of age [106] and most of them are of metastatic origin, particularly from the gastrointestinal or pancreatobiliary tract associated with pseudomyxoma peritonei [5, 107]. Primary OMCs originate mainly from mucinous benign or borderline tumours, with a small percentage originating from mature cystic teratomas or Brenner tumours with gastrointestinal pattern component [106, 107]. They are more commonly unilateral of large size (>13 cm) with no ovarian surface involvement. On the other hand, metastatic mucinous carcinomas are bilateral, smaller in size and associated with pseudomyxoma peritonei and imaging findings from other organs, mainly gastrointestinal or pancreatobiliary tract. They have a favourable prognosis in early clinical stages, albeit in advanced stages they show chemoresistance with unfavourable clinical outcomes [108, 109].

5.1 Pathology of ovarian mucinous carcinomas

Ovarian mucinous carcinomas are usually unilateral masses, large in size (8–40 cm), with the presence of unilocular or multilocular cysts filled with mucinous content. These tumours may display a variety of lesions from cystadenoma areas to borderline mucinous tumour regions and carcinomatous components. Microscopically there are two major histotypes, the intestinal and the endocervical. The intestinal type is more common than the endocervical. They exhibit glandular, cribriform, papillary and solid patterns of growth with two different patterns of invasion (i) expansile/confluent (more common) with a back-to-back glands labyrinthine complex appearance and minimal stroma and (ii) infiltrative/destructive characterised by irregular malignant glands infiltrating desmoplastic stroma. Each pattern of invasion measures 5 mm or more in linear size and they may coexist [5, 108]. Rarely, mural nodules of anaplastic carcinoma or high-grade sarcomatous-like component may be seen in ovarian mucinous carcinomas [5, 110]. There is no standardised grading system for OMCs till now.

5.2 Immunophenotypic features of ovarian mucinous carcinomas

Immunohistochemistry of OMCs is characterised by diffuse intense positivity for CK7 and variable positivity for CA19-9, CEA, CK20 and CDX2 focal weak positivity for PAX8 can be seen in a subset of tumours [111, 112], whereas WT1, Napsin A, Vimentin, CA125, ER and PgR are mostly negative. SATB2 is rarely expressed in ovarian mucinous tumours (5–7%) and its expression is associated with the presence of mature teratoma [113] p53 may demonstrate wild-type or mutation-type immunoreactivity and p16 is usually negative or focally positive [114, 115].

5.3 Molecular pathology of ovarian mucinous carcinomas

OMCs are characterised by *KRAS* and *TP53* mutations (64–66%), *CDKN2A* inactivation (76%) and *HER2/neu* gene amplification (20–26%) [107, 116]. *HER2* gene amplification is almost mutually exclusive to *KRAS* mutations and is found in most of the cases with mutated *TP53* [64%) [116]. OMCs can be developed from benign mucinous tumours through a progression tumour evolution model starting with *KRAS* or *CDKN2A* genomic alterations. Both *KRAS* and *CDKN2A* mutations along with extra genomic copy number aberrations have been found in mucinous borderline tumours and, therefore, are regarded as early molecular events [117, 118]. Chromosomal locus 9p13.3 amplification and *TP53* mutations are identified at the final evolutionary steps of OMCs' progressive carcinogenesis [118]. Other less frequently mutated genes in MOCs are *PIK3CA, PTEN*, *BRAF*, *CTNNB1/APC* (regulators of the β-catenin/Wnt signal transduction pathway), *RNF43* and *ARID1A* (8–12%) [107]. About 34% of

OMCs have neither *KRAS* nor *HER2* gene alterations and are considered to be neoplasms arising from mature cystic teratomas and correlated with an increased risk of recurrence and poor clinical outcome [119]. OMCs with high number of genomic aberrations and mutational burden are associated with high grade and unfavourable prognosis [107]. Targeted therapeutic approaches against *HER2* amplification and/or *MAPK* pathway mutations might be applied along with other inhibitors, such as HDAC inhibitor for *ARID1A,* for more effective tailored treatment of OMCs [120].

6. Ovarian clear cell carcinomas (OCCCs)

Ovarian clear cell carcinomas comprise 10–12% of ovarian carcinomas with relatively high prevalence in young women of East Asian origin [121]. They are frequently associated with endometriosis lesions (50–74% of the cases) and/or clear cell benign (adenofibroma) or borderline tumours, pathologic entities with *PIK3CA* and *ARID1A* precursor genetic alterations [122]. They present mostly as unilateral mass in clinical stage I or II [5] and are considered a high-grade malignancy, although stage I patients have a favourable prognosis. Advanced-stage patients are related to poor clinical outcomes due to chemoresistance. Predisposition risk factors are late menopause, Lynch syndrome and expression of the genetic locus *HNF1B* through epigenetic mechanisms [122]. Lynch syndrome-associated OCCCs or tumours with MMR deficiency are correlated with long survival due to putative tumour immunogenicity [123].

6.1 Pathology of ovarian clear cell carcinomas

Grossly, OCCCs are large (mean size 13 cm) unilateral masses, solid and cystic in appearance, frequently containing endometriosis lesions. Microscopically, they have solid, tubulocystic and papillary architectural patterns and are composed of neoplastic cells characterised as polygonal, cuboidal or hobnail-like cells with clear cytoplasm, atypical nuclei and distinct nucleoli, without prominent pleomorhism [5, 122]. Mitotic activity is less than 5 mitoses per 10 high power fields. The clear cytoplasm is glycogen rich, PAS positive and diastase sensitive. Stromal hyalinization and myxoid appearance can be seen frequently [5].

6.2 Immunophenotypic features of ovarian clear cell carcinomas

OCCCs are strongly immunopositive for Napsin A (80–85%) and HNF1β (80–92%) [124, 125] and negative for WT1, ER and PgR. In addition, OCCCs show a wild-type pattern of p53 expression [126]. Differential diagnosis of OCCCs should be made among ECs and HGSCs because in bothtumours clear cell change can be observed, HGSCs demonstrate positive immunoreaction for WT1 and ER while ECs show positivity for ER [127]. Additionally, both tumours (HGSCs and ECs) are negative for napsin and HNF1β [127].

6.3 Molecular pathology ovarian clear cell carcinomas

The genomic aberrations found in OCCCs involve *PIK3CA* activating mutations (40–50%), *ARID1A* loss of function mutations (50–75%), *MET* gene amplifications, mutations in *ARID1B* (10%), *KRAS* (15%), *PPP2R1A* (15%), *TERT* promoter (15%), *SMARCA4*, *PTEN* (1–5%), *PIK3CA*, *PIK3R1*, *AKT2*, *TP53* (5–20%) and *ZNF217* transcription factor overexpression, which is associated with poor outcome [128, 129]. *PIK3CA* mutations commonly coexist with *ARID1A* genomic alterations and are more frequent in endometriosis-associated OCCCs [128]. Studies on genes involved in antioxidant cell machineries such as *GPX3* (glutathione peroxidase 3), *GLRX3* (glutaredoxin) and *SOD3* (superoxide dismutase) have shown that these genes are highly expressed in CCOCs resulting in tumour chemotherapy resistance [129, 130]. *HER2* gene amplification (15%) and Mismatch Repair (MMR) gene deficiency (2–3%) have also been identified [131]. MMR germline mutations can be found in 10% of OCCCs and may predispose them in developing OCCCs [131]. Therefore, MMR gene expression should be tested by immunohistochemical methods or by MSI testing in order to identify OCCCs associated with MMR deficiency and/or Lynch syndrome. This is important, taking into account that MMR deficient OCCCs are correlated with favourable clinical outcome even in advanced stages [132]. Mutations of the *TP53* gene are usually rare, albeit abnormal p53 expression (7%) has been reported and is associated with adverse prognosis [132]. Molecules involved in the PIK3/AKT/mTOR pathway and loss of function of *ARID1A* gene might be targeted therapeutically by using mTOR inhibitors and through inhibition of EZH2 transcription factor, respectively [133].

Author details

Gabriela-Monica Stanc, Efthymia Souka and Christos Valavanis*
Department of Pathology, Molecular Pathology Unit, 'Metaxa' Cancer Hospital, Piraeus, Greece

*Address all correspondence to: cvalapath@yahoo.com

References

[1] Reid BM, Permuth JB, Sellers TA. Epidemiology of ovarian cancer: A review. Cancer Biology & Medicine. 2017;**14**(1):9-32

[2] Torre LA, Trabert B, DeSantis CE, Miller KD, Samimi G, Runowicz CD, et al. Ovarian cancer statistics, 2018. CA: A Cancer Journal for Clinicians. 2018;**68**(4):284-296

[3] Cancer statistics-Ovarian Cancer 2011-2017. Available from: https://seer.cancer.gov/statfacts/html/ovary.html

[4] Romero I, Leskelä S, Mies BP, Velasco AP, Palacios J. Morphological and molecular heterogeneity of epithelial ovarian cancer: Therapeutic implications. EJC Supplements. 2020;**15**:1-15

[5] WHO Classification of Tumors Editorial Board. WHO Classification of Tumours: Female Genital Tumours. 5th ed. Vol. 4. Lyon (France): International Agency for Research on Cancer; 2020

[6] Prat J, D'Angelo E, Espinosa I. Ovarian carcinomas: At least five different diseases with distinct histological features and molecular genetics. Human Pathology. 2018;**80**:11-27

[7] Kurman RJ, IeM S. The dualistic model of ovarian carcinogenesis: Revisited, revised, and expanded. The American Journal of Pathology. 2016;**186**(4):733-747

[8] Králíčková M, Laganà AS, Ghezzi F, Vetvicka V. Endometriosis and risk of ovarian cancer: What do we know? Archives of Gynecology and Obstetrics. 2020;**301**(1):1-10

[9] Hatina J, Boesch M, Sopper S, Kripnerova M, Wolf D, Reimer D, et al. Ovarian cancer stem cell heterogeneity. Advances in Experimental Medicine and Biology. 2019;**1139**:201-221

[10] Shih IM, Wang Y, Wang TL. The origin of ovarian cancer species and precancerous landscape. The American Journal of Pathology. 2021;**191**(1):26-39

[11] Li HX, Lu ZH, Shen K, Cheng WJ, Malpica A, Zhang J, et al. Advances in serous tubal intraepithelial carcinoma: Correlation with high grade serous carcinoma and ovarian carcinogenesis. International Journal of Clinical and Experimental Pathology. 2014;**7**(3):848-857

[12] Kuhn E, Wang TL, Doberstein K, Bahadirli-Talbott A, Ayhan A, Sehdev AS, et al. CCNE1 amplification and centrosome number abnormality in serous tubal intraepithelial carcinoma: Further evidence supporting its role as a precursor of ovarian high-grade serous carcinoma. Modern Pathology. 2016;**29**(10):1254-1261

[13] Soong TR, Howitt BE, Horowitz N, Nucci MR, Crum CP. The fallopian tube, "precursor escape" and narrowing the knowledge gap to the origins of high-grade serous carcinoma. Gynecologic Oncology. 2019;**152**(2):426-433

[14] Rhyasen GW, Yao Y, Zhang J, Dulak A, Castriotta L, Jacques K, et al. BRD4 amplification facilitates an oncogenic gene expression program in high-grade serous ovarian cancer and confers sensitivity to BET inhibitors. PLoS One. 2018;**13**(7):e0200826

[15] Sehdev AS, Kurman RJ, Kuhn E, IeM S. Serous tubal intraepithelial carcinoma upregulates markers associated with high-grade serous carcinomas including

Rsf-1 (HBXAP), cyclin E and fatty acid synthase. Modern Pathology. 2010;**23**(6):844-855

[16] Ayhan A, Mao TL, Seckin T, Wu CH, Guan B, Ogawa H, et al. Loss of ARID1A expression is an early molecular event in tumor progression from ovarian endometriotic cyst to clear cell and endometrioid carcinoma. International Journal of Gynecological Cancer. 2012;**22**(8):1310-1315

[17] Bulun SE, Wan Y, Matei D. Epithelial mutations in endometriosis: Link to ovarian cancer. Endocrinology. 2019;**160**(3):626-638

[18] Ruderman R, Pavone ME. Ovarian cancer in endometriosis: An update on the clinical and molecular aspects. Minerva Ginecologica. 2017;**69**(3):286-294

[19] Ramalingam P. Morphologic, immunophenotypic, and molecular features of epithelial ovarian cancer. Oncology (Williston Park, N.Y.). 2016;**30**(2):166-176

[20] Prahm KP, Karlsen MA, Høgdall E, Scheller NM, Lundvall L, Nedergaard L, et al. The prognostic value of dividing epithelial ovarian cancer into type I and type II tumors based on pathologic characteristics. Gynecologic Oncology. 2015;**136**(2):205-211

[21] Koshiyama M, Matsumura N, Konishi I. Recent concepts of ovarian carcinogenesis: Type I and type II. BioMed Research International. 2014;**2014**:934261. DOI: 10.1155/2014/934261

[22] Lisio MA, Fu L, Goyeneche A, Gao ZH, Telleria C. High-grade serous ovarian cancer: Basic sciences, clinical and therapeutic standpoints. International Journal of Molecular Sciences. 2019;**20**(4):952

[23] Minion LE, Dolinsky JS, Chase DM, Dunlop CL, Chao EC, Monk BJ. Hereditary predisposition to ovarian cancer, looking beyond BRCA1/BRCA2. Gynecologic Oncology. 2015;**137**(1):86-92

[24] Suszynska M, Ratajska M, Kozlowski P. BRIP1, RAD51C, and RAD51D mutations are associated with high susceptibility to ovarian cancer: Mutation prevalence and precise risk estimates based on a pooled analysis of ~30,000 cases. Journal of Ovarian Research. 2020;**13**(1):50

[25] Chandrasekaran D, Sobocan M, Blyuss O, Miller RE, Evans O, Crusz SM, et al. Implementation of multigene germline and parallel somatic genetic testing in epithelial ovarian cancer: SIGNPOST study. Cancers (Basel). 2021;**13**(17):4344

[26] Soslow RA, Han G, Park KJ, Garg K, Olvera N, Spriggs DR, et al. Morphologic patterns associated with BRCA1 and BRCA2 genotype in ovarian carcinoma. Modern Pathology. 2012;**25**(4):625-636

[27] De Leo A, Santini D, Ceccarelli C, Santandrea G, Palicelli A, Acquaviva G, et al. What is new on ovarian carcinoma: Integrated morphologic and molecular analysis following the new 2020 world health organization classification of female genital tumors. Diagnostics (Basel). 2021;**11**(4):697

[28] Manu V, Hein TA, Boruah D, Srinivas V. Serous ovarian tumors: Immunohistochemical profiling as an aid to grading and understanding tumorigenesis. Medical Journal, Armed Forces India. 2020;**76**(1):30-36

[29] Köbel M, Piskorz AM, Lee S, Lui S, LePage C, Marass F, et al. Optimized p53 immunohistochemistry is an accurate predictor of TP53 mutation in ovarian carcinoma. The Journal of Pathology. Clinical Research. 2016;**2**(4):247-258

[30] Chen M, Yao S, Cao Q, Xia M, Liu J, He M. The prognostic value of Ki67 in ovarian high-grade serous carcinoma: An 11-year cohort study of Chinese patients. Oncotarget. 2016;**8**(64):107877-107885

[31] Ordóñez NG. Value of immunohistochemistry in distinguishing peritoneal mesothelioma from serous carcinoma of the ovary and peritoneum: A review and update. Advances in Anatomic Pathology. 2006;**13**(1):16-25

[32] Köbel M, Ronnett BM, Singh N, Soslow RA, Gilks CB, McCluggage WG. Interpretation of P53 immunohistochemistry in endometrial carcinomas: Toward increased reproducibility. International Journal of Gynecological Pathology. 2019;**38**(1):S123-S131

[33] Al-Hussaini M, Stockman A, Foster H, McCluggage WG. WT-1 assists in distinguishing ovarian from uterine serous carcinoma and in distinguishing between serous and endometrioid ovarian carcinoma. Histopathology. 2004;**44**(2):109-115

[34] Hashi A, Yuminamochi T, Murata S, Iwamoto H, Honda T, Hoshi K. Wilms tumor gene immunoreactivity in primary serous carcinomas of the fallopian tube, ovary, endometrium, and peritoneum. International Journal of Gynecological Pathology. 2003;**22**(4):374-377

[35] Waldstrøm M, Grove A. Immunohistochemical expression of Wilms tumor gene protein in different histologic subtypes of ovarian carcinomas. Archives of Pathology & Laboratory Medicine. 2005;**129**(1):85-88

[36] Wojnarowicz PM, Oros KK, Quinn MC, Arcand SL, Gambaro K, Madore J, et al. The genomic landscape of TP53 and p53 annotated high grade ovarian serous carcinomas from a defined founder population associated with patient outcome. PLoS One. 2012;**7**(9):e45484

[37] Vang R, Levine DA, Soslow RA, Zaloudek C, IeM S, Kurman RJ. Molecular alterations of TP53 are a defining feature of ovarian high-grade serous carcinoma: A rereview of cases lacking TP53 mutations in the cancer genome atlas ovarian study. International Journal of Gynecological Pathology. 2016;**35**(1):48-55

[38] Otsuka I. Mechanisms of high-grade serous carcinogenesis in the fallopian tube and ovary: Current hypotheses, etiologic factors, and molecular alterations. International Journal of Molecular Sciences. 2021;**22**(9):4409

[39] Brown LA, Irving J, Parker R, Kim H, Press JZ, Longacre TA, et al. Amplification of EMSY, a novel oncogene on 11q13, in high grade ovarian surface epithelial carcinomas. Gynecologic Oncology. 2006;**100**(2):264-270

[40] Ballabio S, Craparotta I, Paracchini L, Mannarino L, Corso S, Pezzotta MG, et al. Multisite analysis of high-grade serous epithelial ovarian cancers identifies genomic regions of focal and recurrent copy number alteration in 3q26.2 and 8q24.3. International Journal of Cancer. 2019;**145**(10):2670-2681

[41] Moschetta M, George A, Kaye SB, Banerjee S. BRCA somatic mutations and epigenetic BRCA modifications in serous ovarian cancer. Annals of Oncology. 2016;**27**(8):1449-1455

[42] Takaya H, Nakai H, Takamatsu S, Mandai M, Matsumura N. Homologous recombination deficiency status-based classification of high-grade serous ovarian carcinoma. Scientific Reports. 2020;**10**(1):2757. DOI: 10.1038/s41598-020-59671-3

[43] Pietragalla A, Arcieri M, Marchetti C, Scambia G, Fagotti A. Ovarian cancer predisposition beyond BRCA1 and BRCA2 genes. International Journal of Gynecological Cancer. 2020;**30**(11):1803-1810

[44] Ritterhouse LL, Nowak JA, Strickland KC, Garcia EP, Jia Y, Lindeman NI, et al. Morphologic correlates of molecular alterations in extrauterine Müllerian carcinomas. Modern Pathology. 2016;**29**(8):893-903

[45] Banerjee SN, Lord CJ. First-line PARP inhibition in ovarian cancer - Standard of care for all? Nature Reviews. Clinical Oncology. 2020;**17**(3):136-137

[46] Jiang X, Li X, Li W, Bai H, Zhang Z. PARP inhibitors in ovarian cancer: Sensitivity prediction and resistance mechanisms. Journal of Cellular and Molecular Medicine. 2019;**23**(4):2303-2313

[47] Miller RE, Leary A, Scott CL, Serra V, Lord CJ, Bowtell D, et al. ESMO recommendations on predictive biomarker testing for homologous recombination deficiency and PARP inhibitor benefit in ovarian cancer. Annals of Oncology. 2020;**31**:12, 1606-1622

[48] Sztupinszki Z, Diossy M, Borcsok J, Prosz A, Cornelius N, Kjeldsen MK, et al. Comparative assessment of diagnostic homologous recombination deficiency-associated mutational signatures in ovarian cancer. Clinical Cancer Research. 2021;**27**(20):5681-5687

[49] Stover EH, Fuh K, Konstantinopoulos PA, Matulonis UA, Liu JF. Clinical assays for assessment of homologous recombination DNA repair deficiency. Gynecologic Oncology. 2020;**159**(3):887-898

[50] Weigelt B, Comino-Méndez I, de Bruijn I, Tian L, Meisel JL, García-Murillas I, et al. Diverse BRCA1 and BRCA2 reversion mutations in circulating cell-free DNA of therapy-resistant breast or ovarian cancer. Clinical Cancer Research. 2017;**23**(21):6708-6720

[51] Norquist B, Wurz KA, Pennil CC, Garcia R, Gross J, Sakai W, et al. Secondary somatic mutations restoring BRCA1/2 predict chemotherapy resistance in hereditary ovarian carcinomas. Journal of Clinical Oncology. 2011;**29**(22):3008-3015

[52] Sheta R, Bachvarova M, Plante M, Renaud MC, Sebastianelli A, Gregoire J, et al. Development of a 3D functional assay and identification of biomarkers, predictive for response of high-grade serous ovarian cancer (HGSOC) patients to poly-ADP ribose polymerase inhibitors (PARPis): targeted therapy. Journal of Translational Medicine. 2020;**18**(1):439

[53] Fuh K, Mullen M, Blachut B, Stover E, Konstantinopoulos P, Liu J, et al. Homologous recombination deficiency real-time clinical assays, ready or not? Gynecologic Oncology. 2020;**159**(3):877-886

[54] Konecny GE, Wang C, Hamidi H, Winterhoff B, Kalli KR, Dering J, et al. Prognostic and therapeutic relevance of molecular subtypes in high-grade serous ovarian cancer. Journal of the National Cancer Institute. 2014;**106**(10):dju249

[55] Cook DP, Vanderhyden BC. Ovarian cancer and the evolution of subtype classifications using transcriptional profiling†. Biology of Reproduction. 2019;**101**(3):645-658

[56] Mota A, Oltra S, S, Moreno-Bueno G. Insight updating of the molecular

hallmarks in ovarian carcinoma. EJC Supplements. 2020;**15**:16-26

[57] Wang C, Cicek MS, Charbonneau B, Kalli KR, Armasu SM, Larson MC, et al. Tumor hypomethylation at 6p21.3 associates with longer time to recurrence of high-grade serous epithelial ovarian cancer. Cancer Research. 2014;**74**(11):3084-3091

[58] Bodelon C, Killian JK, Sampson JN, Anderson WF, Matsuno R, Brinton LA, et al. Molecular classification of epithelial ovarian cancer based on methylation profiling: Evidence for survival heterogeneity. Clinical Cancer Research. 2019;**25**(19):5937-5946

[59] Li J, Wang J, Chen R, Bai Y, Lu X. The prognostic value of tumor-infiltrating T lymphocytes in ovarian cancer. Oncotarget. 2017;**8**(9):15621-15631

[60] Wang L. Prognostic effect of programmed death-ligand 1 (PD-L1) in ovarian cancer: A systematic review, meta-analysis and bioinformatics study. Journal of Ovarian Research. 2019;**12**(1):37

[61] Darb-Esfahani S, Kunze CA, Kulbe H, Sehouli J, Wienert S, Lindner J, et al. Prognostic impact of programmed cell death-1 (PD-1) and PD-ligand 1 (PD-L1) expression in cancer cells and tumor-infiltrating lymphocytes in ovarian high grade serous carcinoma. Oncotarget. 2016;**7**(2):1486-1499

[62] Whitehair R, Peres LC, Mills AM. Expression of the immune checkpoints LAG-3 and PD-L1 in high-grade serous ovarian carcinoma: Relationship to tumor-associated lymphocytes and germline BRCA status. International Journal of Gynecological Pathology. 2020;**39**(6):558-566

[63] Huang CC, Cheng SH, Wu CH, Li WY, Wang JS, Kung ML, et al. Delta-like 1 homologue promotes tumorigenesis and epithelial-mesenchymal transition of ovarian high-grade serous carcinoma through activation of Notch signaling. Oncogene. 2019;**38**(17):3201-3215

[64] Chen S, Cavazza E, Barlier C, Salleron J, Filhine-Tresarrieu P, Gavoilles C, et al. Beside P53 and PTEN: Identification of molecular alterations of the RAS/MAPK and PI3K/AKT signaling pathways in high-grade serous ovarian carcinomas to determine potential novel therapeutic targets. Oncology Letters. 2016;**12**(5):3264-3272

[65] Pfisterer J, Du Bois A, Bentz EK, Kommoss F, Harter P, Huober J, et al. Prognostic value of human epidermal growth factor receptor 2 (Her-2)/neu in patients with advanced ovarian cancer treated with platinum/paclitaxel as first-line chemotherapy: A retrospective evaluation of the AGO-OVAR 3 Trial by the AGO OVAR Germany. International Journal of Gynecological Cancer. 2009;**19**(1):109-115

[66] Ersoy E, Cao QJ, Otis CN. HER2 protein overexpression and gene amplification in tubo-ovarian high-grade serous carcinomas. International Journal of Gynecological Pathology. 2022;**41**(4):313-319

[67] Slomovitz B, Gourley C, Carey MS, Malpica A, Shih IM, Huntsman D, et al. Low-grade serous ovarian cancer: State of the science. Gynecologic Oncology. 2020;**156**(3):715-725

[68] Longacre TA, McKenney JK, Tazelaar HD, Kempson RL, Hendrickson MR. Ovarian serous tumors of low malignant potential (borderline tumors): Outcome-based study of 276 patients with long-term (> or =5-year) follow-up. The American Journal of Surgical Pathology. 2005;**29**(6): 707-723

[69] Bell DA. Low-grade serous tumors of ovary. International

Journal of Gynecological Pathology. 2014;**33**(4):348-356

[70] O'Neill CJ, Deavers MT, Malpica A, Foster H, McCluggage WG. An immunohistochemical comparison between low-grade and high-grade ovarian serous carcinomas: Significantly higher expression of p53, MIB1, BCL2, HER-2/neu, and C-KIT in high-grade neoplasms. The American Journal of Surgical Pathology. 2005;**29**(8):1034-1041

[71] Van Nieuwenhuysen E, Busschaert P, Laenen A, Moerman P, Han SN, Neven P, et al. Loss of 1p36.33 frequent in low-grade serous ovarian cancer. Neoplasia. 2019;**21**(6):582-590

[72] Hunter SM, Anglesio MS, Ryland GL, Sharma R, Chiew YE, Rowley SM, et al. Molecular profiling of low grade serous ovarian tumours identifies novel candidate driver genes. Oncotarget. 2015;**6**(35):37663-37677

[73] Anglesio MS, Arnold JM, George J, Tinker AV, Tothill R, Waddell N, et al. Mutation of ERBB2 provides a novel alternative mechanism for the ubiquitous activation of RAS-MAPK in ovarian serous low malignant potential tumors. Molecular Cancer Research. 2008;**6**(11):1678-1690

[74] Ho CL, Kurman RJ, Dehari R, Wang TL, IeM S. Mutations of BRAF and KRAS precede the development of ovarian serous borderline tumors. Cancer Research. 2004;**64**(19):6915-6918

[75] Tsang YT, Deavers MT, Sun CC, Kwan SY, Kuo E, Malpica A, et al. KRAS (but not BRAF) mutations in ovarian serous borderline tumour are associated with recurrent low-grade serous carcinoma. The Journal of Pathology. 2013;**231**(4):449-456

[76] Grisham RN, Iyer G, Garg K, Delair D, Hyman DM, Zhou Q, et al. BRAF mutation is associated with early stage disease and improved outcome in patients with low-grade serous ovarian cancer. Cancer. 2013;**119**(3):548-554

[77] Zyla RE, Olkhov-Mitsel E, Amemiya Y, Bassiouny D, Seth A, Djordjevic B, et al. CTNNB1 mutations and aberrant β-catenin expression in ovarian endometrioid carcinoma: Correlation with patient outcome. The American Journal of Surgical Pathology. 2021;**45**(1):68-76

[78] Farley J, Brady WE, Vathipadiekal V, Lankes HA, Coleman R, Morgan MA, et al. Selumetinib in women with recurrent low-grade serous carcinoma of the ovary or peritoneum: An open-label, single-arm, phase 2 study. The Lancet Oncology. 2013;**14**(2):134-140

[79] Nasioudis D, Latif NA, Simpkins F, Cory L, Giuntoli RL 2nd, Haggerty AF, et al. Adjuvant chemotherapy for early stage endometrioid ovarian carcinoma: An analysis of the National Cancer Data Base. Gynecologic Oncology. 2020;**156**(2):315-319

[80] Terada T. Endometrioid adenocarcinoma of the ovary arising in atypical endometriosis. International Journal of Clinical and Experimental Pathology. 2012;**5**(9):924-927

[81] Helder-Woolderink JM, Blok EA, Vasen HF, Hollema H, Mourits MJ, De Bock GH. Ovarian cancer in Lynch syndrome; a systematic review. European Journal of Cancer. 2016;**55**:65-73

[82] Assem H, Rambau PF, Lee S, Ogilvie T, Sienko A, Kelemen LE, et al. High-grade endometrioid carcinoma of the ovary: A clinicopathologic study of 30 cases. The American Journal of Surgical Pathology. 2018;**42**(4):534-544

[83] Santandrea G, Piana S, Valli R, Zanelli M, Gasparini E, De Leo A, et al. Immunohistochemical biomarkers as a surrogate of molecular analysis in ovarian carcinomas: A review of the literature. Diagnostics (Basel). 2021;**11**(2):199

[84] Köbel M, Rahimi K, Rambau PF, Naugler C, Le Page C, Meunier L, et al. An immunohistochemical algorithm for ovarian carcinoma typing. International Journal of Gynecological Pathology. 2016;**35**(5):430-441

[85] Chiarelli S, Buriticá C, Litta P, Ciani S, Guarch R, Nogales FF. An immunohistochemical study of morules in endometrioid lesions of the female genital tract: CD10 is a characteristic marker of morular metaplasia. Clinical Cancer Research. 2006;**12**(14 Pt 1): 4251-4256

[86] Houghton O, Connolly LE, McCluggage WG. Morules in endometrioid proliferations of the uterus and ovary consistently express the intestinal transcription factor CDX2. Histopathology. 2008;**53**(2):156-165

[87] Lim D, Murali R, Murray MP, Veras E, Park KJ, Soslow RA. Morphological and immunohistochemical reevaluation of tumors initially diagnosed as ovarian endometrioid carcinoma with emphasis on high-grade tumors. The American Journal of Surgical Pathology. 2016;**40**(3):302-312

[88] Wiegand KC, Shah SP, Al-Agha OM, Zhao Y, Tse K, Zeng T, et al. ARID1A mutations in endometriosis-associated ovarian carcinomas. The New England Journal of Medicine. 2010;**363**(16):1532-1543

[89] Samartzis EP, Noske A, Dedes KJ, Fink D, Imesch P. ARID1A mutations and PI3K/AKT pathway alterations in endometriosis and endometriosis-associated ovarian carcinomas. International Journal of Molecular Sciences. 2013;**14**(9):18824-18849

[90] Oliva E, Sarrió D, Brachtel EF, Sánchez-Estévez C, Soslow RA, Moreno-Bueno G, et al. High frequency of beta-catenin mutations in borderline endometrioid tumours of the ovary. The Journal of Pathology. 2006;**208**(5):708-713

[91] Cybulska P, Paula ADC, Tseng J, Leitao MM Jr, Bashashati A, Huntsman DG, et al. Molecular profiling and molecular classification of endometrioid ovarian carcinomas. Gynecologic Oncology. 2019;**154**(3):516-523

[92] Leskela S, Romero I, Rosa-Rosa JM, Caniego-Casas T, Cristobal E, Pérez-Mies B, et al. Molecular heterogeneity of endometrioid ovarian carcinoma: An analysis of 166 cases using the endometrial cancer subrogate molecular classification. The American Journal of Surgical Pathology. 2020;**44**(7):982-990

[93] Leskela S, Romero I, Cristobal E, Pérez-Mies B, Rosa-Rosa JM, Gutierrez-Pecharroman A, et al. Mismatch repair deficiency in ovarian carcinoma: Frequency, causes, and consequences. The American Journal of Surgical Pathology. 2020;**44**(5):649-656

[94] Bennett JA, Pesci A, Morales-Oyarvide V, Da Silva A, Nardi V, Oliva E. Incidence of mismatch repair protein deficiency and associated clinicopathologic features in a cohort of 104 ovarian endometrioid carcinomas. The American Journal of Surgical Pathology. 2019;**43**(2):235-243

[95] Hollis RL, Thomson JP, Stanley B, Churchman M, Meynert AM, Rye T, et al.

Molecular stratification of endometrioid ovarian carcinoma predicts clinical outcome. Nature Communications. 2020;**11**(1):4995

[96] Chui MH, Ryan P, Radigan J, Ferguson SE, Pollett A, Aronson M, et al. The histomorphology of Lynch syndrome-associated ovarian carcinomas: Toward a subtype-specific screening strategy. The American Journal of Surgical Pathology. 2014;**38**(9):1173-1181

[97] Wang L, Rambau PF, Kelemen LE, Anglesio MS, Leung S, Talhouk A, et al. Nuclear β-catenin and CDX2 expression in ovarian endometrioid carcinoma identify patients with favourable outcome. Histopathology. 2019;**74**(3):452-462

[98] Brett MA, Atenafu EG, Singh N, Ghatage P, Clarke BA, Nelson GS, et al. Equivalent survival of p53 mutated endometrial endometrioid carcinoma grade 3 and endometrial serous carcinoma. International Journal of Gynecological Pathology. 2021;**40**(2):116-123

[99] Anglesio MS, Wang YK, Maassen M, Horlings HM, Bashashati A, Senz J, et al. Synchronous endometrial and ovarian carcinomas: Evidence of clonality. Journal of the National Cancer Institute. 2016;**108**(6):djv428

[100] Schultheis AM, Ng CK, De Filippo MR, Piscuoglio S, Macedo GS, Gatius S, et al. Massively parallel sequencing-based clonality analysis of synchronous endometrioid endometrial and ovarian carcinomas. Journal of the National Cancer Institute. 2016;**108**(6):djv427

[101] Kurman RJ, Shih IM. Seromucinous tumors of the ovary. What's in a Name? International Journal of Gynecological Pathology. 2016;**35**(1):78-81

[102] Ben-Mussa A, McCluggage WG. Ovarian seromucinous cystadenomas and adenofibromas: First report of a case series. Histopathology. 2021;**78**(3):445-452

[103] Parra-Herran C, Lerner-Ellis J, Xu B, Khalouei S, Bassiouny D, Cesari M, et al. Molecular-based classification algorithm for endometrial carcinoma categorizes ovarian endometrioid carcinoma into prognostically significant groups. Modern Pathology. 2017;**30**(12):1748-1759

[104] Fukumoto T, Park PH, Wu S, Fatkhutdinov N, Karakashev S, Nacarelli T, et al. Repurposing Pan-HDAC inhibitors for ARID1A-mutated ovarian cancer. Cell Reports. 2018;**22**(13):3393-3400

[105] Lee JM, Minasian L, Kohn EC. New strategies in ovarian cancer treatment. Cancer. 2019;**125**(Suppl. 24):4623-4629

[106] Babaier A, Ghatage P. Mucinous cancer of the ovary: Overview and current status. Diagnostics (Basel). 2020;**10**(1):52

[107] Cheasley D, Wakefield MJ, R yland GL, Allan PE, Alsop K, Amarasinghe KC, et al. The molecular origin and taxonomy of mucinous ovarian carcinoma. Nature Communications. 2019;**10**(1):3935

[108] Gouy S, Saidani M, Maulard A, Bach-Hamba S, Bentivegna E, Leary A, et al. Characteristics and prognosis of stage i ovarian mucinous tumors according to expansile or infiltrative type. International Journal of Gynecological Cancer. 2018;**28**(3):493-499

[109] Hada T, Miyamoto M, Ishibashi H, Matsuura H, Sakamoto T, Kakimoto S, et al. Survival and biomarker analysis

for ovarian mucinous carcinoma according to invasive patterns: Retrospective analysis and review literature. Journal of Ovarian Research. 2021;**14**(1):33

[110] Provenza C, Young RH, Prat J. Anaplastic carcinoma in mucinous ovarian tumors: A clinicopathologic study of 34 cases emphasizing the crucial impact of stage on prognosis, their histologic spectrum, and overlap with sarcomalike mural nodules. The American Journal of Surgical Pathology. 2008;**32**(3):383-389

[111] Vang R, Gown AM, Barry TS, Wheeler DT, Yemelyanova A, Seidman JD, et al. Cytokeratins 7 and 20 in primary and secondary mucinous tumors of the ovary: Analysis of coordinate immunohistochemical expression profiles and staining distribution in 179 cases. The American Journal of Surgical Pathology. 2006;**30**(9):1130-1139

[112] Vang R, Gown AM, Wu LS, Barry TS, Wheeler DT, Yemelyanova A, et al. Immunohistochemical expression of CDX2 in primary ovarian mucinous tumors and metastatic mucinous carcinomas involving the ovary: Comparison with CK20 and correlation with coordinate expression of CK7. Modern Pathology. 2006;**19**(11):1421-1428

[113] Schmoeckel E, Kirchner T, Mayr D. SATB2 is a supportive marker for the differentiation of a primary mucinous tumor of the ovary and an ovarian metastasis of a low-grade appendiceal mucinous neoplasm (LAMN): A series of seven cases. Pathology, Research and Practice. 2018;**214**(3):426-430

[114] McCluggage WG. Immunohistochemistry in the distinction between primary and metastatic ovarian mucinous neoplasms. Journal of Clinical Pathology. 2012;**65**(7):596-600

[115] Tabrizi AD, Kalloger SE, Köbel M, Cipollone J, Roskelley CD, Mehl E, et al. Primary ovarian mucinous carcinoma of intestinal type: Significance of pattern of invasion and immunohistochemical expression profile in a series of 31 cases. International Journal of Gynecological Pathology. 2010;**29**(2):99-107

[116] Anglesio MS, Kommoss S, Tolcher MC, Clarke B, Galletta L, Porter H, et al. Molecular characterization of mucinous ovarian tumours supports a stratified treatment approach with HER2 targeting in 19% of carcinomas. The Journal of Pathology. 2013;**229**(1):111-120

[117] Hunter SM, Gorringe KL, Christie M, Rowley SM, Bowtell DD, Australian Ovarian Cancer Study Group, et al. Pre-invasive ovarian mucinous tumors are characterized by CDKN2A and RAS pathway aberrations. Clinical Cancer Research. 2012;**18**(19):5267-5277

[118] Mackenzie R, Kommoss S, Winterhoff BJ, Kipp BR, Garcia JJ, Voss J, et al. Targeted deep sequencing of mucinous ovarian tumors reveals multiple overlapping RAS-pathway activating mutations in borderline and cancerous neoplasms. BMC Cancer. 2015;**15**:415

[119] Bouri S, Simon P, D'Haene N, Catteau X, Noël JC. P53 and PIK3CA Mutations in KRAS/HER2 negative ovarian intestinal-type mucinous carcinoma associated with mature teratoma. Case Reports in Obstetrics and Gynecology. 2020;**2020**:8863610

[120] Gorringe KL, Cheasley D, Wakefield MJ, Ryland GL, Allan PE, Alsop K, et al. Therapeutic options for mucinous ovarian carcinoma.

Gynecologic Oncology. 2020;**156**(3): 552-560

[121] Liu H, Xu Y, Ji J, Dong R, Qiu H, Dai X. Prognosis of ovarian clear cell cancer compared with other epithelial cancer types: A population-based analysis. Oncology Letters. 2020;**19**(3):1947-1957

[122] Iida Y, Okamoto A, Hollis RL, Gourley C, Herrington CS. Clear cell carcinoma of the ovary: A clinical and molecular perspective. International Journal of Gynecological Cancer. 2021;**31**(4):605-616

[123] Stewart CJ, Bowtell DD, Doherty DA, Leung YC. Long-term survival of patients with mismatch repair protein-deficient, high-stage ovarian clear cell carcinoma. Histopathology. 2017;**70**(2):309-313

[124] Skirnisdottir I, Bjersand K, Akerud H, Seidal T. Napsin A as a marker of clear cell ovarian carcinoma. BMC Cancer. 2013;**13**:524

[125] Li Q, Zeng X, Cheng X, Zhang J, Ji J, Wang J, et al. Diagnostic value of dual detection of hepatocyte nuclear factor 1 beta (HNF-1β) and napsin A for diagnosing ovarian clear cell carcinoma. International Journal of Clinical and Experimental Pathology. 2015;**8**(7):8305-8310

[126] Heckl M, Schmoeckel E, Hertlein L, Rottmann M, Jeschke U, Mayr D. The ARID1A, p53 and ß-Catenin statuses are strong prognosticators in clear cell and endometrioid carcinoma of the ovary and the endometrium. PLoS One. 2018;**13**(2):e0192881

[127] Köbel M, Kalloger SE, Carrick J, Huntsman D, Asad H, Oliva E, et al. A limited panel of immunomarkers can reliably distinguish between clear cell and high-grade serous carcinoma of the ovary. The American Journal of Surgical Pathology. 2009;**33**(1):14-21

[128] Huang HN, Lin MC, Huang WC, Chiang YC, Kuo KT. Loss of ARID1A expression and its relationship with PI3K-Akt pathway alterations and ZNF217 amplification in ovarian clear cell carcinoma. Modern Pathology. 2014;**27**(7):983-990

[129] Friedlander ML, Russell K, Millis S, Gatalica Z, Bender R, Voss A. Molecular profiling of clear cell ovarian cancers: identifying potential treatment targets for clinical trials. International Journal of Gynecological Cancer. 2016;**26**(4):648-654

[130] Takano M, Tsuda H, Sugiyama T. Clear cell carcinoma of the ovary: Is there a role of histology-specific treatment? Journal of Experimental & Clinical Cancer Research. 2012;**31**(1):53

[131] Bennett JA, Morales-Oyarvide V, Campbell S, Longacre TA, Oliva E. Mismatch repair protein expression in clear cell carcinoma of the ovary: Incidence and morphologic associations in 109 cases. The American Journal of Surgical Pathology. 2016;**40**(5):656-663

[132] Parra-Herran C, Bassiouny D, Lerner-Ellis J, Olkhov-Mitsel E, Ismiil N, Hogen L, et al. Mismatch repair protein, and POLE abnormalities in ovarian clear cell carcinoma: An outcome-based clinicopathologic analysis. The American Journal of Surgical Pathology. 2019;**43**(12):1591-1599

[133] Bitler BG, Aird KM, Garipov A, Li H, Amatangelo M, Kossenkov AV, et al. Synthetic lethality by targeting EZH2 methyltransferase activity in ARID1A-mutated cancers. Nature Medicine. 2015;**21**(3):231-238

Section 2

Tumour Angiogenesis in Ovarian Cancer

Chapter 3

Role of Human Epididymis Protein 4 in Tumour Angiogenesis

Harshita Dubey, Mansi Modi, Saransh Verma, Ruchi Sinha, Harsh Goel, Amar Ranjan, Pranay Tanwar, Anita Chopra, Ekta Rahul, Lawanya Ranjan, Neeraj Verma, Devender Singh Chauhan, Rani Kumari Mahkam and Utkarsh Dubey

Abstract

HE4 is a secretory protein. It is expressed in reproductive tract and respiratory epithelium in normal individuals. Serum level of HE4 is raised in various solid cancers that give us an advantage to use it as a diagnostic and prognostic biomarker. It is an established biomarker of epithelial ovarian cancer [EOC]. It has also shown the significance in various other malignancies like cancer of endometrium, cervix, lung and breast. Studies show HE4 as an independent prognostic biomarker in non-small cell lung carcinoma. Its raised values in cancer signify its role in oncogenesis. HE4 promotes angiogenesis via STAT3 signalling pathway. In this paper we have tried to illustrate about human epididymis protein 4 and its role in tumour angiogenesis.

Keywords: HE4, tumour angiogenesis, oncogenesis, HIF1a, ovary

1. Introduction

Ovarian cancer is one of the most common gynaecologic malignancies that have the highest mortality rate. Ovarian cancer is the third most common [after cervical and corpus uteri] gynaecological malignancy worldwide and it is the most deadly gynaecological malignancy [1]. The disease produces few and nonspecific symptoms early in the course of illness. Consequently about 70% of the cases are diagnosed in the advanced stage [stage 3 and 4] with a 5 year survival of less than 30%. The disease has a good prognosis if diagnosed in the early stages, with a 5 year survival rate in stage 1 disease being 83.4–89.6% [2].

Therefore it is imperative to diagnose the disease early to improve prognosis and reduce mortality.

Diagnosis is usually based on clinical examination followed by transvaginal ultrasonography. Both these methods suffer from low specificity and subjectivity and are thus not recommended for screening.

The differentiation between benign and malignant ovarian disease is often only possible after histological examination of the resected ovarian tissue. It subjects the women to unnecessary surgical procedures which could be avoided if reliable, accurate, noninvasive tests were to become available as a majority of ovarian masses in both premenopausal and postmenopausal women are benign.

This is followed by measurement of serum biomarker levels the most common being CA125, and HE4. Though CA125 is an established biomarker, it has a low specificity and can be elevated in other benign gynaecological conditions and malignancies. 40–50% patients with epithelial ovarian cancer [EOC's] have normal CA125 levels [3].

HE4 is the only other biomarker approved by FDA for monitoring response to treatment and recurrence of disease in EOC. HE4 is a secretory protein of the whey acidic protein [WAP] family. The expression of HE4 is restricted to reproductive tract and respiratory epithelium in normal individuals. HE4 levels are over expressed in EOC tissues and serves as a sensitive and specific serum marker for diagnosis, prognosis and disease recurrence. It is also less likely to be elevated in benign conditions. HE4 levels may also be elevated in other malignancies such as endometrial cancer and pulmonary neoplasms and has been proposed as a biomarker for these conditions [4].

2. Expression of HE4 in tumours

HE4 is a secretory glycoprotein. It is over-expressed in ovarian carcinomas especially in serous and endometriod variants. It is also called whey-acidic-protein that belongs to WAP domain family. WAP is a four-disulfide core domain protein 2 [WFDC2]. It was initially described to have tissue specific expression in epididymis [5].

Available literature revealed that HE4 is expressed in female reproductive tract, breast tissue, kidney, regions of the respiratory tract and nasopharynx [6–8]. Moreover, it is also expressed in normal human trachea, salivary glands, lung, prostate, pituitary gland, thyroid, and kidney [8]. It's an independent prognostic marker in non-small cell lung cancer [NSCLC] [9].

3. HE4 as a biomarker in ovarian cancer

HE4 is a complementary biomarker to CA125 (Carbohydrates Antigen125). HE4 has potential to complement or even is a better alternative to carbohydrate antigen 125 (CA125) [10–12]. Currently CA125 is being used as a biomarker for the diagnosis and therapeutic monitoring in ovarian cancer. CA125 is raised in only 50% of stage I epithelial ovarian cancers, and only about 80% in all epithelial ovarian cancers [13]. So for all practical purposes, CA125 cannot be used as an independent biomarkerfor the diagnosis of EOC, while HE4 can be used as a stand-alone biomarker, in both diagnosis and prognosis of EOC and endometrial cancers [14, 15]. It has also been approved by the United States of America (USA), Food and Drug Administration (FDA) as a biomarker to monitor patients with epithelial ovarian cancer [16].

Studies show that serum level of HE4 and CA125 together can be used as an indicator of prognosis in ovarian cancer. The two together has shown positive results, sensitivity of 76.4% and specificity of 95% [17]. Individually, HE4 is a well known biomarker for the diagnosis and therapeutic monitoring for ovarian cancer.

4. Role of HE4 in the pathogenesis of ovarian cancer

HE4 is also involved in the pathogenesis of ovarian cancer. It aids in cellular proliferation, tumour growth, metastatic ability, chemoresistance and suppresses cytotoxic effect of mononuclear cells on ovarian carcinoma cells [18]. An inverse relationship between serum HE4 levels and CD8+ T cells in EOC has also been noted [19, 20].

Angiogenesis is one of the hallmarks of cancer and is necessary for bringing oxygen and nutrients to tumour cells and removal of waste products. It aids in tumour growth and invasion [21].

Hypoxia inducible factor 1 alpha (HIF1a) is a transcription factor that is involved in adaptation of cells to a hypoxic environment through its pro-angiogenic actions.

Interleukin 8 (IL-8) is also an important pro angiogenic factor produced by infiltrating macrophages in the tumour. Both of these factors are up-regulated by STAT3.

Recent studies have shown that HE4 promotes angiogenesis and is dependent on intact STAT3 signalling for its action. The addition of STAT3 inhibitors ablated elevated HIF1a levels in an in vitro experiment involving ovarian cancer cell lines and also blocked tube formation in human umbilical vein endothelial cell [19].

Several patients of ovarian cancer experience a chemo resistant recurrence within 2 years after first line therapy (cytoreduction surgery and platinum based chemotherapeutics) [18].

The diverse effects of HE4 that aid in tumour progression makes it an attractive therapeutic target for EOC and may serve as a effective treatment option for recurrent chemoresistant cases.

HE4 is produced as a, 13 kDa protein and converted to a, 25 kDa secreted glycosylated protein. HE4 is a highly over-expressed in epithelial ovarian cancer (EOC) [15, 22–24] compared to normal ovarian epithelium. US-FDA has approved HE4 as a biomarker for the diagnosis of ovarian cancer especially in the presence of an adnexal mass as part of the Risk of Ovarian Malignancy Algorithm (ROMA) [2].

5. Mechanism of action of HE4 in angiogenesis

Angiogenetic function of HE4 is promoted by epidermal growth factor (EGF), vascular endothelial growth factor (VEGF) and insulin. EGF & VEGF works through nuclear translocation, while insulin works through nucleolar translocation. EGF, VEGF and Insulin along with their receptors promotes tumour growth and proliferation in ovarian cancer [25–27]. VEGF is essential for hypoxia-inducible factor mediated neo-vascularisation and it is regulated by the hypoxia-inducible factor (HIF) family [28].

HE4 leads to the activation of protein STAT3, which gets phosphorylated by the receptor associated with Janus Kinases (JAK). It promotes translocation in the nucleus. Here it acts as a transcription activator.

The growth and proliferation of tumour cells leads to local hypoxia and inflammation leading to the activation of STAT3 to produce factors that promotes angiogenesis. VEGF is a potent proangiogenic factor that helps endothelial cells to induce angiogenesis. The signal from VEGF stimulates STAT3 that is responsible for endothelial cell proliferation. It also induces metaststic activity of tumour cells by regulating the transcription of the targeted genes.

Furthermore, STAT3 signalling promotes the up-regulation of pro-angiogenic STAT3 target genes IL8 and HIF1A in immune cells, ovarian cancer cells, and endothelial cells. Moreover, HE4 promotes increase in tube formation in an *in vitro* model of angiogenesis, which is also dependent upon STAT3 signalling.

Firstly, the rapid proliferation of tumour cells leads to local hypoxia and inflammation, which activate STAT3 in tumour cells to produce pro-angiogenic factor. Further, VEGF (vascular endothelial growth factor) is a potent pro- angiogenic factor which promotes endothelial cell angiogenesis. The VEGF signal activates STAT3 which subsequently promotes endothelial cell proliferation and migration by regulating the transcription of the targeted genes.

Furthermore, STAT3 signalling promotes the up-regulation of pro-angiogenic STAT3 target genes IL8 and HIF1A in immune cells, ovarian cancer cells, and endothelial cells. Moreover, HE4 promotes increase in tube formation in an *in vitro* model of angiogenesis, which is also dependent upon STAT3 signalling.

Clinically, the positive correlation has been seen in between the serum levels of HE4 and IL8 in ovarian cancer patients. HE4 has been shown to be associated with microvascular density ovarian cancer tissue. HE4 is also shown to be inversely correlated with the amount of cytotoxic T cell infiltration. These phenomena suggest that HE4 may cause deregulated vascular proliferation and it suppresses T cell trafficking in tumour tissues [29].

HE4 has potential to alter the signalling pathways to modify the expression of related gene in the tumour micro-environment. Thus it affects angiogenesis and immunogenic responses in especially in ovarian cancer [29].

Tumour angiogenesis is also regulated by programmed cell death-1 (PD-1) that suppresses the anti-tumour function of CD8 + T cells [30].

The tumour vasculature is also regulated by the cytokines secreted by immune cells, and an interlinked activities have been studied between angiogenesis and immune suppression [31]. Human epididymis protein 4 (HE4) also functions as anti-proteases [5, 6]. It inhibits the cytotoxic activities of mononuclear cells in the tumour micro-environment of ovarian cancer cells [7, 32].

HE4 promotes oncogenesis in ovarian cancer not only by promoting cell proliferation, metastasis, and chemo resistance, but it also by altering the tumour microenvironment. Because of being secretory protein, HE4 can function as intracellularly or by autocrine or paracrine mechanisms [1].

The angiogenesis mediated by immune cells is regulated through the activation of STAT3, which is mediated by HE4. STAT3 is responsible for immune suppression solid tumours [33–35]. The inhibitor T cell receptor ligand PD-L1 is also associated with tumour angiogenesis. It is regulated by HIF1α (Hypoxia-induciblefactor1-alpha) through transcription [36]. HIF1α binds to the HE4 gene promoter to up-regulate its transcription [37]. IL8 is a potent pro-angiogenic factor. Its expression is one of the poor prognostic factors of high-grade serous ovarian cancer [38]. HIF1α has also shown to promote angiogenesis and alters the metabolic environment in cancer [39, 40].

6. Role of HE4 in tumorigenesis

HE4 promotes tumorigenesis through its pro-angiogenic effects. Various studies have shown the role of HE4 in tumour angiogenesis. HE4 modulates angiogenesis by regulating the expression of different genes in multiple cell types of the tumour environment [19]. HE4 activates protein kinase B (AKT) which plays a role in tumour angiogenesis [41, 42]. James et al. have shown that HE4 activates signal transducer and activator of transcription 3 (STAT3) signalling pathway which up-regulates the pro-angiogenic genes interleukin 8 (IL8), hypoxia inducible factor 1A (HIF1A) in ovarian cancer cells, endothelial cells, and immune cells [19, 42, 43]. Levels of both HE4 and the pro-angiogenic factors were found elevated in ovarian cancer tissue in comparison to adjacent normal ovarian tissue [19, 42]. IL8 and HIF1A are potent angiogenic factors that promote tumour vessel formation and tumour growth [42]. IL8 also leads to persistent neutrophil recruitment in the tumour tissue which stimulates neoangiogenesis [44, 45]. HIF1A plays a role in hypoxic adaptation of cancer cells [46, 47]. STAT3 inhibitors block the effect of HE4- mediated tube formation of endothelium by suppressing STAT3 activation and down-regulating IL8 and HIF1A [19]. HE4 has been shown to be associated with increased levels of matrix metalloproteinases which are responsible for angiogenesis [48, 49]. Levels of HE4 and interleukin-1 alpha (IL1A) are directly proportional [50, 51]. IL1A promotes VEGF formation [52]. Annexin II (ANXA2) too is involved in angiogenesis and its gene expression has been increased by HE4 [53]. HE4 has also been found to promote tube formation in in-vitro model of angiogenesis [19]. Serum levels of HE4 positively correlated with the microvascular density in ovarian cancer tissue as reflected by the increased CD34+ areas in the tumour tissue. However, the new vessel formation is dysregulated [19]. These dysfunctional tumoral vasculature impair the movement of cytotoxic T cells along with other immune cells involved in host's anti-tumour immune responses [54].

7. Prognostic and predictive value of HE4 in ovarian cancer

Presently, there is no predictive biomarker for the success of chemotherapy. Studies show that HE4 and CA 125 values become negative after fourth cycle chemotherapy if there is a good response. Rise in HE4 is seen earlier than CA 125. Long term progression-free survival is associated with the serum levels of biomarker lower than the mean value in the affected population at the time of diagnosis and the development of negativity of the marker after third cycle of chemotherapy. Monitoring of HE4 and Ca125 during chemotherapy especially after third cycle is recommended for their prognostic values [55].

8. Conclusion

HE4, a secretory glycoprotein is over-expressed in ovarian cancer most commonly in the serous and endometriod variants. It is a complementary biomarker to CA125. When HE is used in combination with CA125, the diagnostic and prognostic performance of ovarian cancer is increased significantly. HE4 is involved in oncogenesis by promoting cellular growth, proliferation, metastasis and chemoresistance in ovarian cancer. HIF1a and Interleukin 8 are associated pro-angiogenetic factors, which are up-regulated by STAT3 pathway. Angiogenetic action of HE4 is also associated with epidermal growth factor, vascular endothelial growth factor (VEGF) and insulin which promoted nuclear translocations. So, research on HE4 may decode some novel mechanisms of oncogenesis to provide alternative therapeutic options.

Conflict of interest

"The authors declare no conflict of interest".

Author details

Harshita Dubey[1], Mansi Modi[2], Saransh Verma[1], Ruchi Sinha[1], Harsh Goel[1], Amar Ranjan[1*], Pranay Tanwar[1], Anita Chopra[1], Ekta Rahul[1], Lawanya Ranjan[3], Neeraj Verma[4], Devender Singh Chauhan[5], Rani Kumari Mahkam[6] and Utkarsh Dubey[7]

1 All India Institute of Medical Sciences, New Delhi, India

2 Hindu Rao Hospital, Delhi, India

3 Monash College, Melbourne, Australia

4 Lady Hardinge Medical College, New Delhi, India

5 ABV Institute of Medical Sciences, New Delhi, India

6 Sanjeevan Hospital, New Delhi, India

7 AD Institute of Technology and Management, Delhi, India

*Address all correspondence to: dr.amarranjan@rediffmail.com

References

[1] Momenimovahed Z, Tiznobaik A, Taheri S, Salehiniya H. Ovarian cancer in the world: Epidemiology and risk factors. International Journal of Women's Health. 2019;**11**:287-299

[2] Heintz A, Odicino F, Maisonneuve P, Quinn MA, Benedet JL, Creasman WT, et al. Carcinoma of the ovary. International Journal of Gynecology and Obstetrics. Nov 2006;**95**(Suppl 1):S161-S192. DOI: 10.1016/S0020-7292(06)60033-7. PMID: 29644669

[3] Scaletta G, Plotti F, Luvero D, Capriglione S, Montera R, Miranda A, et al. The role of novel biomarker HE4 in the diagnosis, prognosis and follow-up of ovarian cancer: A systematic review. Expert Review of Anticancer Therapy. 2017;**17**(9):827-839

[4] Moore RG, Miller MC, Steinhoff MM, Skates SJ, Lu KH, Lambert-Messerlian G, et al. Serum HE4 levels are less frequently elevated than CA125 in women with benign gynecologic disorders. American Journal of Obstetrics and Gynecology. 2012;**206**(4):351.e1-351.e8

[5] Kirchhoff C, Habben I, Ivell R, Krull N. A major human epididymis-specific cDNA encodes a protein with sequence homology to extracellular proteinase inhibitors1. Biology of Reproduction. 1991;**45**(2):350-357

[6] Bingle L, Singleton V, Bingle CD. The putative ovarian tumour marker gene HE4 (WFDC2), is expressed in normal tissues and undergoes complex alternative splicing to yield multiple protein isoforms. Oncogene. 18 Apr 2002;**21**(17):2768-2773. DOI: 10.1038/sj.onc.1205363. PMID: 11965550

[7] James NE, Oliver MT, Ribeiro JR, Cantillo E, Rowswell-Turner RB, Kim KK, et al. Human epididymis secretory protein 4 (HE4) compromises cytotoxic mononuclear cells via inducing dual specificity phosphatase 6. Frontiers in Pharmacology. 19 Mar 2019;**10**:216. DOI: 10.3389/fphar.2019.00216. PMID: 30941033; PMCID: PMC6433991

[8] Galgano MT, Hampton GM, Frierson HF Jr. Comprehensive analysis of HE4 expression in normal and malignant human tissues. Modern Pathology. Jun 2006;**19**(6):847-853. DOI: 10.1038/modpathol.3800612. PMID: 16607372

[9] Lamy PJ, Plassot C, Pujol JL. Serum HE4: An independent prognostic factor in non-small cell lung cancer. PLoS One. 1 Jun 2015;**10**(6):e0128836. DOI: 10.1371/journal.pone.0128836. PMID: 26030627; PMCID: PMC4452338

[10] Kalapotharakos G, Asciutto C, Henic E, et al. High preoperative blood levels of HE4 predicts poor prognosis in patients with ovarian cancer. Journal of Ovarian Research. 2012;**5**:20. DOI: 10.1186/1757-2215-5-20

[11] Hamed EO, Ahmed H, Sedeek OB, Mohammed AM, Abd-Alla AA, Abdel Ghaffar HM. Significance of HE4 estimation in comparison with CA125 in diagnosis of ovarian cancer and assessment of treatment response. Diagnostic Pathology. 23 Jan 2013;**8**:11. DOI: 10.1186/1746-1596-8-11. PMID: 23343214; PMCID: PMC3621278

[12] Molina R, Escudero JM, Augé JM, Filella X, Foj L, Torné A, et al. HE4 a novel tumour marker for ovarian cancer: Comparison with CA 125 and ROMA algorithm in patients with gynaecological diseases. Tumor Biology. Dec 2011;32(6):1087-1095. DOI: 10.1007/s13277-011-0204-3. Epub 2011 Aug 24. PMID: 21863264; PMCID: PMC3195682

[13] Zurawski VR Jr, Knapp RC, Einhorn N, Kenemans P, Mortel R, Ohmi K, et al. An initial analysis of preoperative serum CA 125 levels in patients with early stage ovarian carcinoma. Gynecologic Oncology. May 1988;**30**(1):7-14. DOI: 10.1016/0090-8258(88)90039-x. PMID: 2452773

[14] Mutz-Dehbalaie I, Egle D, Fessler S, Hubalek M, Fiegl H, Marth C, et al. HE4 is an independent prognostic marker in endometrial cancer patients. Gynecologic Oncology. 1 Aug 2012;**126**(2):186-191

[15] Hellström I, Raycraft J, Hayden-Ledbetter M, Ledbetter JA, Schummer M, McIntosh M, et al. The HE4 (WFDC2) protein is a biomarker for ovarian carcinoma. Cancer Research. 1 Jul 2003;**63**(13):3695-3700. PMID: 12839961

[16] Bandiera E, Romani C, Specchia C, Zanotti L, Galli C, Ruggeri G, et al. Serum human epididymis protein 4 and risk for ovarian malignancy algorithm as new diagnostic and prognostic tools for epithelial ovarian cancer management. Cancer Epidemiology, Biomarkers & Prevention. Dec 2011;**20**(12):2496-2506

[17] Moore RG, Brown AK, Miller MC, Skates S, Allard WJ, Verch T, et al. The use of multiple novel tumor biomarkers for the detection of ovarian carcinoma in patients with a pelvic mass. Gynecologic Oncology. 1 Feb 2008;**108**(2):402-408

[18] James NE, Chichester C, Ribeiro JR. Beyond the biomarker: Understanding the diverse roles of human epididymis protein 4 in the pathogenesis of epithelial ovarian cancer. Frontiers in Oncology. 24 Apr 2018;**8**:124

[19] James NE, Emerson JB, Borgstadt AD, Beffa L, Oliver MT, Hovanesian V, et al. The biomarker HE4 (WFDC2) promotes a pro-angiogenic and immunosuppressive tumor microenvironment via regulation of STAT3 target genes. Scientific Reports. 2020;**10**:8558

[20] Zhu L, Zhuang H, Wang H, Tan M, Schwab CL, Deng L, et al. Overexpression of HE4 (human epididymis protein 4) enhances proliferation, invasion and metastasis of ovarian cancer. Oncotarget. 2016;7(1):729-744

[21] Folkman J. Angiogenesis in cancer, vascular, rheumatoid and other disease. Nature Medicine. 1995;**1**(1):27-30

[22] Ono K, Tanaka T, Tsunoda T, Kitahara O, Kihara C, Okamoto A, et al. Identification by cDNA microarray of genes involved in ovarian carcinogenesis. Cancer Research. 15 Sep 2000;**60**(18):5007-5011. PMID: 11016619

[23] Welsh JB, Zarrinkar PP, Sapinoso LM, Kern SG, Behling CA, Monk BJ, et al. Analysis of gene expression profiles in normal and neoplastic ovarian tissue samples identifies candidate molecular markers of epithelial ovarian cancer. Proceedings of the National Academy of Sciences of the United States of America. 30 Jan 2001;**98**(3):1176-1181. DOI: 10.1073/pnas.98.3.1176. PMID: 11158614; PMCID: PMC14728

[24] Huhtinen K, Suvitie P, Hiissa J, Junnila J, Huvila J, Kujari H, et al. Serum HE4 concentration differentiates malignant ovarian tumours from ovarian endometriotic cysts. British Journal of Cancer. 21 Apr 2009;**100**(8):1315-1319. DOI: 10.1038/sj.bjc.6605011. Epub 2009 Mar 31. PMID: 19337252; PMCID: PMC2676558

[25] Poddar A, Aranha RR, Muthukaliannan KG, Nachimuthu R, Jayaraj R. Head and neck cancer risk

factors in India: Protocol for systematic review and meta-analysis. BMJ Open. 20 Aug 2018;**8**(8):e020014. DOI: 10.1136/bmjopen-2017-020014. PMID: 30127047; PMCID: PMC6104749

[26] Karna H, Gonzalez J, Radia HS, Sedghizadeh PP, Enciso R. Risk-reductive dental strategies for medication related osteonecrosis of the jaw among cancer patients: A systematic review with meta-analyses. Oral Oncology. 1 Oct 2018;**85**:15-23

[27] Jayaraj R, Kumarasamy C, Madurantakam Royam M, Devi A, Baxi S. Is HIF-1α a viable prognostic indicator in OSCC? A critical review of a meta-analysis study. World Journal of Surgical Oncology. Dec 2018;**16**(1):1-2

[28] Tam S, Fu S, Xu L, Krause KJ, Lairson DR, Miao H, et al. The epidemiology of oral human papillomavirus infection in healthy populations: A systematic review and meta-analysis. Oral oncology. 1 Jul 2018;**82**:91-99

[29] James NE, Emerson JB, Borgstadt AD, Beffa L, Oliver MT, Hovanesian V, et al. The biomarker HE4 (WFDC2) promotes a pro-angiogenic and immunosuppressive tumor microenvironment via regulation of STAT3 target genes. Scientific Reports. 22 May 2020;**10**(1):8558. DOI: 10.1038/s41598-020-65353-x. PMID: 32444701; PMCID: PMC7244765

[30] Zhang G, Liu C, Bai H, Cao G, Cui R, Zhang Z. Combinatorial therapy of immune checkpoint and cancer pathways provides a novel perspective on ovarian cancer treatment. Oncology Letters. 1 Mar 2019;**17**(3):2583-2591

[31] Shi JU, Wei PK. Interleukin-8: A potent promoter of angiogenesis in gastric cancer. Oncology letters. 1 Feb 2016;**11**(2):1043-1050

[32] James NE, Cantillo E, Oliver MT, Rowswell-Turner RB, Ribeiro JR, Kim KK, et al. HE4 suppresses the expression of osteopontin in mononuclear cells and compromises their cytotoxicity against ovarian cancer cells. Clinical & Experimental Immunology. Sep 2018;**193**(3):327-340

[33] Chang N, Ahn SH, Kong DS, Lee HW, Nam DH. The role of STAT3 in glioblastoma progression through dual influences on tumor cells and the immune microenvironment. Molecular and Cellular Endocrinology. 2017;**451**:53-65

[34] Tkach M, Coria L, Rosemblit C, Rivas MA, Proietti CJ, DíazFlaqué MC, et al. Targeting Stat3 induces senescence in tumor cells and elicits prophylactic and therapeutic immune responses against breast cancer growth mediated by NK cells and CD4+ T cells. Journal of Immunology. 1 Aug 2012;**189**(3):1162-1172

[35] Liu JF, Deng WW, Chen L, Li YC, Wu L, Ma SR, et al. Inhibition of JAK2/STAT3 reduces tumor-induced angiogenesis and myeloid-derived suppressor cells in head and neck cancer. Molecular Carcinogenesis. Mar 2018;**57**(3):429-439

[36] Chen J, Jiang CC, Jin L, Zhang XD. Regulation of PD-L1: A novel role of pro-survival signalling in cancer. Annals of Oncology. 1 Mar 2016;**27**(3):409-416

[37] Peng C, Liu G, Huang K, Zheng Q, Li Y, Yu C. Hypoxia-induced upregulation of HE4 is responsible for resistance to radiation therapy of gastric cancer. Molecular Therapy-Oncolytics. 29 Mar 2019;**12**:49-55

[38] Sanguinete MM, Oliveira PH, Martins-Filho A, Micheli DC, Tavares-Murta BM, Murta EF, et al. Serum IL-6 and IL-8 correlate with

prognostic factors in ovarian cancer. Immunological investigations. 3 Oct 2017;**46**(7):677-688

[39] Choi SH, Kwon OJ, Park JY, Kim DY, Ahn SH, Kim SU, et al. Inhibition of tumour angiogenesis and growth by small hairpin HIF-1α and IL-8 in hepatocellular carcinoma. Liver International. Apr 2014;**34**(4):632-642

[40] Regulation of angiogenesis by hypoxia: Role of the HIF system. Nature Medicine [Internet]. 2022. Available from: https://www.nature.com/articles/nm0603-677

[41] Lee S, Choi S, Lee Y, Chung D, Hong S, Park N. Role of human epididymis protein 4 in chemoresistance and prognosis of epithelial ovarian cancer. Journal of Obstetrics and Gynaecology Research. Jan 2017;**43**(1):220-227

[42] Ribeiro JR, Schorl C, Yano N, Romano N, Kim KK, Singh RK, et al. HE4 promotes collateral resistance to cisplastin and paclitaxel in ovarian cancer cells. Journal of Ovarian Research. 2016;**9**:28

[43] Oka. Signal transducer and activator of transcription 3 upregulates interleukin-8 expression at the level of transcription in human melanoma cells. Experimental Dermatology. 2010. Available from: https://onlinelibrary.wiley.com/doi/full/10.1111/j.1600-0625.2009.00972.x

[44] Fu H et al. Persisting and increasing neutrophil infiltration associates with gastric carcinogenesis and E-cadherin downregulation. Scientific Reports. 2016;**6**:29762. DOI: 10.1038/srep29762

[45] Bekes EM et al. Tumor-recurited neutrophils and neutrophil TIMP-free MMP-9 regulate coordinately the levels of tumor angiogenesis and efficiency of malignant cell intravasation. The American Journal of Pathology. 2011;**179**:1455-1470

[46] Maxwell PH, Wiesener MS, Chang GW, Clifford SC, Vaux EC, Cockman ME, et al. The tumor suppressor protein VHL targets hypoxia-inducible factors for oxygen-dependent proteolysis. Nature. 1999;**399**:271-275

[47] Dang CV, Semenza GL. Oncogenic alterations of metabolism. Trends in Biochemical Sciences. 1999;**24**:68-72

[48] Cathcart J, Pulkoski-Gross A, Cao J. Targeting matrix metalloproteinases in cancer: Bringing new life to old ideas. Genes & Diseases. 2015;**2**:26-34

[49] Lakka SS, Gondi CS, Rao JS. Proteases and glioma angiogenesis. Brain Pathology. 2005;**15**:327-341

[50] Zhu L, Zhuang H, Wang H, Tan M, Schwab CL, Deng L, et al. Overexpression of HE4 (human epididymis protein 4) enhances proliferation, invasion and metastasis of ovaian cancer. Oncotarget. 2015;**7**:729-744

[51] Zhu L, Guo Q, Jin S, Feng H, Zhuang H, Liu C, et al. Analysis of the gene expression profile in response to human epididymis protein 4 in epithelial ovarian cancer cells. Oncology Reports. 2016;**36**:1592-1604

[52] Dabkeviciene D, Sasnauskiene A, Leman E, Kvietkauskaite R, Daugelavicience N, Stankevicius V, et al. MTHPC-mediated photodynamic treatment up-regulates the cytokines VEGF and IL-1 alpha. PhotochemPhotobiol. 2012;**88**:432-439

[53] Zhuang H, Tan M, Liu J, Hu Z, Liu D, Gao J, et al. Human epididymis protein 4

in association with Annexin II promotes invasion and metastasis of ovarian cancer cells. Molecular Cancer. Dec 2014;**13**(1):1-4

[54] Huang Y, Goel S, Duda DG, Fukumura D, Jain RK. Vascular normalization as an emerging strategy to enhance cancer immunotherapy. Cancer Research. 2013;**73**:2943-2948

[55] Potenza E, Parpinel G, Laudani ME, Macchi C, Fuso L, Zola P. Prognostic and predictive value of combined HE-4 and CA-125 biomarkers during chemotherapy in patients with epithelial ovarian cancer. The International Journal of Biological Markers. 2020;**35**(4):20-27

Section 3

Chemoresistance and Ovarian Cancer

Chapter 4

Integrins in Ovarian Cancer: Survival Pathways, Malignant Ascites and Targeted Photochemistry

Mustafa Kemal Ruhi, Brittany P. Rickard, William J. Polacheck and Imran Rizvi

Abstract

Integrins are surface adhesion molecules that, upon binding to ligands, cluster to form adhesion complexes. These adhesion complexes are comprised of structural and regulatory proteins that modulate a variety of cellular behaviors including differentiation, growth, and migration through bidirectional signaling activities. Aberrant integrin expression and activation in ovarian cancer plays a key role in the detachment of cancer cells from primary sites as well as migration, invasion, and spheroid formation. An emerging area is the activation or rearrangement of integrins due to mechanical stress in the tumor microenvironment, particularly in response to fluid shear stress imparted by currents of malignant ascites. This chapter describes the role of integrins in ovarian cancer with an emphasis on crosstalk with survival pathways, the effect of malignant ascites, and discusses the literature on integrin-targeting approaches in ovarian cancer, including targeted photochemistry for therapy and imaging.

Keywords: ovarian cancer, integrins, ascites, photodynamic therapy, targeted photochemistry

1. Introduction

High-grade serous ovarian carcinoma (HGSOC, ovarian cancer) is the most common and most fatal type of gynecologic malignancy. HGSOC accounts for 75% of all epithelial ovarian cancers and for 5% of all cancer deaths [1, 2]. In most cases, HGSOC develops without symptoms and is diagnosed at an advanced stage, when malignant cells are already disseminated within the peritoneal cavity [2, 3]. Metastasis in ovarian cancer commonly occurs via transcoelomic routes, which is associated with cell detachment from the primary tumor site and dissemination as single cells or spheroids, where alterations in cell-cell and cell-extracellular matrix adhesion play a critical role [3–5]. Among the transmembrane adhesion molecules that have altered expression and function in many cancers, including in ovarian cancer, are integrins [6]. In humans, 24 different integrins are formed by specific combinations of 18 α and 8 β non-covalently bound heterodimer subunits [7, 8]. The large extracellular domains of integrins recognize specific amino acid sequences that are found on extracellular matrix (ECM) proteins such as fibronectin, collagen, laminin, and vitronectin. The short cytoplasmic tails in the c-terminus of integrins are linked to the actin cytoskeleton [7, 9]. Upon binding to ligands, integrins cluster to form adhesion complexes, which are comprised of proteins and enzymes that play roles in maintaining bidirectional signaling activities [10, 11]. In "outside-in" signaling, integrins that are bound to ECM ligands activate signaling pathways that lead to cellular responses, including survival and differentiation. Via this physical link, integrins can also transduce signals in a force-dependent manner, when the cell is exposed to mechanical stimuli. In "inside-out" signaling, intracellular conformational changes modulate the affinity of the integrins to ECM ligands [9–13]. Therefore, in addition to cell adhesion, a variety of cellular behaviors including differentiation, growth, and migration, can be mediated by integrins [7, 11]. In cancer, the expression and activation of integrins can be aberrant [14]. Additionally, since the ECM of solid tumors is usually disorganized and the crosslinking of ECM proteins is increased, integrin-mediated signaling is also altered, leading to the progression and drug resistance of the disease [15, 16]. Specifically in ovarian cancer, integrins play a key role in cancer cell detachment, migration, spheroid formation, and invasion, including as a result of the movement of fluid that accumulates within the peritoneal cavity, known as ascites (**Figure 1**) [5].

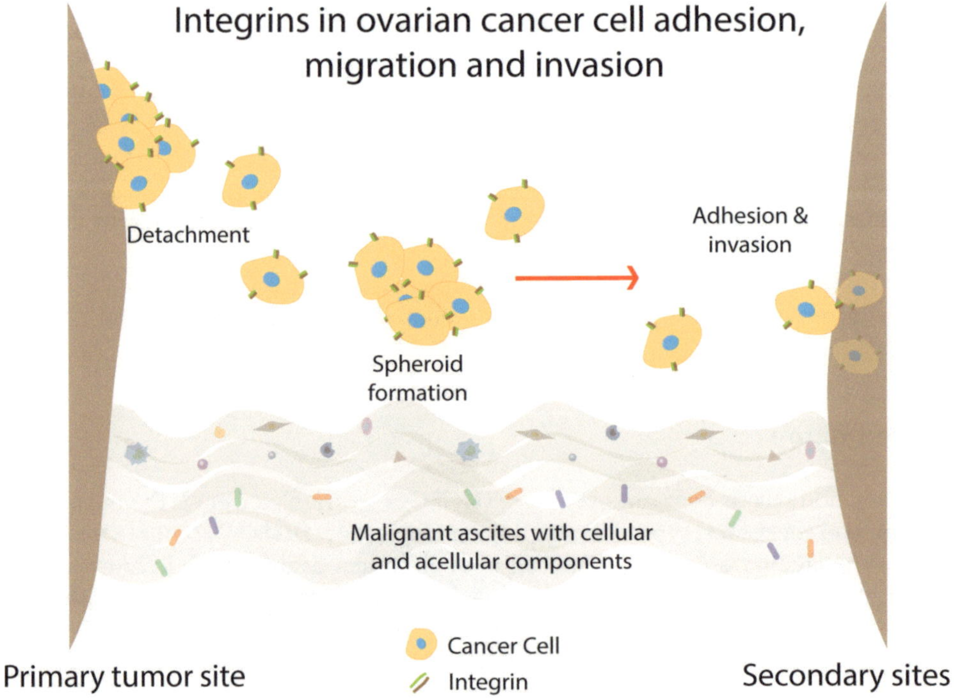

Figure 1.
Integrins play a key role in ovarian cancer progression including cell detachment from primary sites, spheroid formation, migration, adhesion to secondary sites, and invasion.

This review describes the role of integrins in ovarian cancer and discusses the current literature in integrin-targeted approaches for ovarian cancer, including photochemistry-based imaging and therapy.

2. Integrins in ovarian cancer and the significance of ascites

2.1 Integrins and integrin-associated survival pathways in ovarian cancer

The potential role of integrins in critical processes leading to ovarian cancer progression, including the detachment of cancer cells from primary sites, spheroid formation, migration, adhesion to secondary sites, and invasion has been reported by multiple groups [17–28]. The clustering of collagen-binding integrins $\alpha_2\beta_1$ and $\alpha_3\beta_1$ is associated with increased expression and activity of matrix metalloproteinase-9 (MMP-9). An increase in activated MMP-9 is associated with the shedding of E-cadherin, a transmembrane glycoprotein that regulates cell-to-cell adhesion, and increased epithelial-mesenchymal transition (EMT), changes that are indicative of an invasive and metastatic phenotype in ovarian cancer cells [17–20]. The $\alpha_v\beta_6$ integrin has also been associated with protease secretion and ECM degradation in ovarian cancer cell lines, both of which are indicators of invasive potential [21–23]. Collagen-binding integrins, including heterodimer $\alpha_4\beta_1$, have also been implicated in ovarian cancer migration by Slack-Davis *et al.*, who showed that transmigration of SKOV3 cells through a mesothelial monolayer model decreased significantly upon blocking of α_4 integrin, β_1 integrin, or vascular cell adhesion protein-1 (VCAM-1). VCAM-1 is a glycoprotein that is predominantly expressed on endothelial cells, but, under high levels of inflammation and in chronic pathological conditions, is also expressed on other cell types, including macrophages and cancer cells [29]. The aforementioned findings by Slack-Davis *et al.* suggest that the VCAM-1-$\alpha_4\beta_1$ integrin interaction is involved in ovarian cancer cell metastasis and invasion through the mesothelium [24]. In addition to migration and invasive potential, studies have found that α_5 and β_1 integrins are critical for ovarian cancer cell spheroid formation as well as their adhesion to different ligands including fibronectin, laminin and collagen IV, further implicating integrins in ovarian cancer progression [25–28].

In the context of integrins, disease progression, and drug resistance in ovarian cancer, cell signaling pathways, including PI3K/Akt, Ras/Raf/MEK/ERK, Wnt, YAP/TAZ, as well as crosstalk between integrins and the epidermal growth factor receptor (EGFR), have been most commonly investigated (**Figure 2**) [30–35]. A key player in the activation of the aforementioned pathways is focal adhesion kinase (FAK), a tyrosine kinase that localizes to focal adhesions [34, 36–40]. The overexpression of FAK is frequently associated with advanced-stage ovarian cancer and with increased invasiveness [41], thus FAK inhibition has been investigated as a treatment approach for ovarian cancer [42, 43]. The following subsections describe the current state of the literature on integrin-mediated activation of key molecules and survival pathways that contribute to ovarian cancer progression.

2.1.1 PI3K/Akt pathway

The PI3K/Akt pathway transduces signals from the cell membrane to the cytoplasm and mediates fundamental cellular functions including proliferation and survival [44, 45]. Upon activation by a growth factor, receptor tyrosine kinases (RTKs)

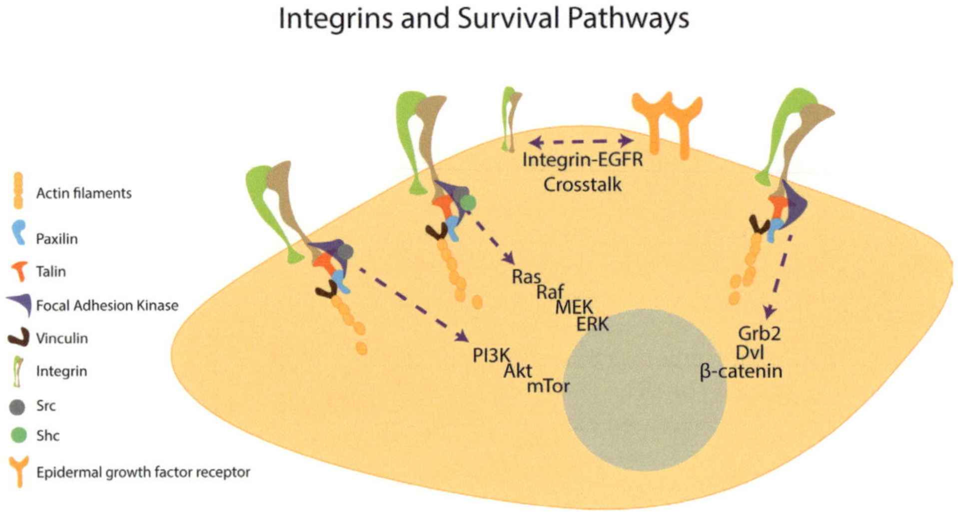

Figure 2.
Integrin activation can influence cell survival pathways: (1) the PI3K/Akt survival pathway involves the recruitment of FAK to focal adhesions. FAK can propagate the PI3K/Akt pathway, either directly or through Src kinase. (2) Shc phosphorylation by both Src and FAK, which initiates the Shc-Grb2-Sos-Ras cascade may lead to ERK phosphorylation. (3) FAK activation by integrins may also lead to the activation of Wnt/β-catenin pathway. Crosstalk between EGFR and integrins can potentiate signaling and cooperatively stimulate intracellular pathways that contribute to cell survival and drug resistance.

activate PI3K and trigger its conversion from phosphatidylinositol-4, 5-bisphosphate (PIP2) to phosphatidylinositol-3, 4, 5-triphosphate (PIP3). The serine/threonine kinase Akt interacts with PIP3, which causes its translocation to the plasma inner membrane, where it is phosphorylated by phosphatidylinositide-dependent kinase 1 (PDK1) and PDK2, known as Ser473-phosphorylated Akt kinase. The phosphorylated and activated Akt may interact with substrates that regulate cell growth and survival, including mTOR, Glycogen synthase kinase-3 (GSK3), Bad, and caspase-9. The PI3K/Akt pathway can also be activated by other cell surface receptors such as cytokine receptors and integrins. A recent study Zheng *et al.*, found that $\alpha_2\beta_1$ overexpressing ($\alpha_2\beta_1^+$) ovarian cancer cells, and ovarian cancer patient tissue samples that were resistant to microtubule-directed chemotherapeutic drugs, including paclitaxel and vincristine, had enhanced PI3K and Akt phosphorylation, as well as Akt translocation into the nucleus [30]. This suggests that $\alpha_2\beta_1$ integrins activate the PI3K/AKT pathway to promote resistance to microtubule-directed chemotherapeutic drugs.

Integrin-mediated activation of PI3K/Akt survival pathway involves the recruitment of FAK to the adhesion complex [36]. FAK interacts with the cytoplasmic tail of β-subunits on integrins and forms a dual kinase complex with c-Src. FAK can activate the PI3K/Akt pathway, either directly or through Src kinase. The relationship between FAK signaling and PI3K/Akt pathway-mediated resistance to taxane-based therapy has been demonstrated in a study Kang *et al*. The authors found that VS-6063, a FAK inhibitor, synergized with paclitaxel in HeyA8-MDR cells and showed an additive inhibitory effect with paclitaxel in the taxane resistant cell lines SKOV3-TR and SKOV3ip1 [42]. Decreased tumor weight was also reported in the same study in mouse models of these cell lines after treatment with paclitaxel and VS-6063 compared to paclitaxel alone. Others have also explored the effectiveness of VS-6063 in ovarian cancer growth inhibition [43]. Xu *et al.* screened combinations of VS-6063 with 30 potent inhibitors and found that JQ1, an inhibitor of the Myc oncogenic network, synergized with VS-6063. Although the efficacy was dependent on the cell line, using VS-6063 and JQ1 caused an additive or synergistic inhibition effect in proliferation and viability of ovarian cancer cells by inhibiting active FAK and c-Myc, as well as their signaling, through the PI3K/Akt pathway.

2.1.2 Ras/Raf/MEK/ERK pathway

The Ras/Raf/MEK/ERK pathway, one of the major signaling cascades of the mitogen-activated protein kinase (MAPK) family, plays a key role in cell proliferation, differentiation, motility, and survival [46], and is dysregulated in one-third of human tumors [47]. Activation of this pathway can occur through a variety of mechanisms, including integrin-mediated cell adhesion or activation of membrane RTKs by extracellular stimuli such as growth factors, hormones, cytokines, and mitogens [48]. Although this pathway can be activated by either cell adhesion or growth factors, strong and sustainable ERK activation results from cooperative signaling by both RTKs and integrins [38, 49]. In RTK-mediated signaling, the activation of RTKs leads to the activation of the small GTP-binding protein Ras. Ras recruits Raf kinases to the cell membrane, which in turn activate MEK1 and MEK2, leading to the phosphorylation of ERK1 and ERK2, catalyzed by MEK. Phosphorylated ERK1 and ERK2 translocate to the nucleus and initiate phosphorylation of transcription factors, such as c-Myc, c-fos, Ets, and Elk1 [47]. In contrast to RTK signaling cascades, integrin-mediated signal transduction in this pathway is less dependent on Ras and is instead initiated by autophosphorylation of FAK and the formation of FAK-Src complexes [39]. According to the model for adhesion-mediated ERK activation suggested by Yee *et al.*, Shc is phosphorylated by both Src and FAK, which initiates the Shc-Grb2-Sos-Ras cascade, leading to ERK phosphorylation [38].

As mentioned above, Shc phosphorylation by FAK and Src is an important step in integrin-mediated activation of the Ras/Raf/MEK/ERK pathway because only some integrins, including $\alpha_1\beta_1$, $\alpha_5\beta_1$, $\alpha_6\beta_4$, and $\alpha_v\beta_3$, can recruit Shc to the FAK-Src complex [50]. Similarly, certain integrins, like $\alpha_v\beta_6$ integrin, play key roles in MEK/ERK activation which can lead to cancer-associated changes in the Ras/Raf/MEK/ERK pathway [31, 32]. Studies have shown that ERK activation, induced by thyroid hormone administration, in high $\alpha_v\beta_3$-expressing ovarian cancer cells enhances cell proliferation and survival, while inhibition of the Ras/Raf/MEK/ERK pathway increased ovarian cancer cell susceptibility to treatment in both chemosensitive and chemoresistant lines [51–54]. In summary, integrin overexpression, notably that of $\alpha_v\beta_3$ and $\alpha_v\beta_6$ integrins, may contribute to ovarian cancer progression and resistance to therapies by promoting activation of the Ras/Raf/MEK/ERK pathway cooperatively with RTK-mediated signaling.

2.1.3 Wnt pathway

Wnt signaling cascades regulate multiple cellular processes including cell polarity, migration, adhesion, proliferation, and developmental events, such as embryogenesis and tissue morphogenesis [33, 55]. The two main Wnt pathways, non-canonical and canonical, are characterized by the involvement of β-catenin, which is one of the key components in cell-cell adhesion and cell migration, in addition to its role in Wnt-mediated gene transcription. In non-canonical signaling, small GTPases of the Rho family or heterotrimeric G proteins, independently from β-catenin, are activated to control cell polarity and calcium signaling, respectively [56, 57]. The Wnt/β-catenin pathway (a.k.a. canonical pathway) is initiated via the activation of the frizzled receptor by Wnt proteins [58]. Activated receptors recruit and activate the cytoplasmic protein Disheveled, which inactivates the β-catenin destruction complex that is composed of proteins, including Axin, Adenomatous Polyposis Coli (APC) and GSK-3β. Since β-catenin levels are kept low by the destruction complex, the inactivation of the complex enables cytoplasmic accumulation of β-catenin. Accumulated β-catenin then translocates to the nucleus and interacts with the TCF/LEF family proteins to control transcription [55, 56].

In cancer, Wnt signaling becomes dysregulated and Wnt target genes can regulate tumor progression and drug resistance [55, 58, 59]. The Wnt/β-catenin pathway is associated with poor prognosis in ovarian tumors and has been shown to be a key regulator of chemoresistance in different cancer types including ovarian, colon, prostate, and pancreatic [60–63]. In a study by Viscarra *et al.*, transcriptomic sequencing analysis of parental and carboplatin-resistant A2780 cells revealed 156 differentially expressed genes, among which those related to the Wnt/β-catenin pathway and integrin signaling were the most enriched (15.2 and 10.9%, respectively) [64]. Upregulation of one of the integrin signaling pathway members, COL11A1, in carboplatin-resistant A2780 cells is important to note because COL11A1 overexpression has been reported to be an indicator of poor prognosis, metastasis, and drug resistance in ovarian cancer. Interestingly, Viscarra *et al.* also reported that, compared to carboplatin-resistant A2780 cells, parental A2780 cells showed significant increases in caspase-3/7 cleavage, which are indicators of apoptosis. Together these findings suggest that integrins and the Wnt/β-catenin pathway can synergistically regulate carboplatin resistance in A2780 cells [64, 65]. In accordance with these findings, a study by Crampton *et al.* revealed that integrin-mediated signals can synergize with the Wnt pathway through the adapter protein growth factor Grb2 [33]. Additionally, Burkhalter *et al.* found that integrin clustering and binding to collagen increased nuclear β-catenin levels, thereby promoting transcriptional activation of Wnt/β-catenin pathway target genes [66].

2.1.4 YAP/TAZ transcriptional regulators

Yes-associated protein 1 (YAP) and Transcriptional coactivator with PDZ-binding motif (TAZ) are two transcriptional regulators that play an important role in mechanotransduction, i.e., converting external mechanical inputs to cellular responses [67]. YAP and TAZ (YAP/TAZ) are known as coactivators in the Hippo pathway, a signaling pathway that plays a role in homeostasis, organ size control, cell differentiation, and the progression of various types of human cancer, including ovarian cancer [68, 69]. Active YAP/TAZ translocates to the nucleus to interact with TEA domain family member (TEAD) transcription factors, where the YAP/TAZ-TEAD protein complex transcribes genes that control cell proliferation and apoptosis [70]. In addition to their role in the Hippo pathway, YAP/TAZ also interact with the Wnt pathway and mediate Wnt signaling [68, 71]. Research has shown that integrins and other components in adhesion complexes, including FAK and Src, can also activate YAP/TAZ to maintain mechanotransduction [40, 72]. The overexpression and activation of YAP/TAZ have been shown to be correlated with poor prognosis in ovarian cancer [73–79]. Specifically, YAP was shown to play an important role in ovarian cancer tumorigenesis, cell proliferation, invasion, and resistance to therapy *in vitro* and *in vivo* [74, 76]. Expression and activation of YAP [76] and TAZ [79] were also associated with poor prognosis and resistance to chemotherapy in tissue samples from ovarian cancer patients. As a result of these findings, the therapeutic potential of YAP/TAZ inhibition in ovarian cancer has become a topic of recent research [75, 80–82]. In summary, the studies discussed above reveal that Wnt signaling pathway and YAP/TAZ, which can be activated by integrins, are key regulators in ovarian cancer invasion and drug resistance.

2.1.5 Epidermal growth factor receptor-integrin crosstalk

EGFR is a cell surface RTK, the activation of which initiates cell proliferation and survival pathways including PI3K/Akt and Ras/Raf/MEK/ERK [83]. High expression of EGFR is associated with an aggressive and invasive phenotype in multiple cancer types including ovarian cancer [84–88]. Interestingly, integrin-mediated ECM adhesion can induce tyrosine phosphorylation of EGFR in the absence of EGF, and if both EGF and activated integrins are present, they can promote sustained EGFR signaling [89, 90]. For example, EGFR expression in OV-MZ-6 cells is correlated with $\alpha_v\beta_3$ integrin levels [34]. In the same cells, the activity of MAPK and FAK was increased upon stimulation of $\alpha_v\beta_3$ integrins and EGFR by vitronectin and EGF, respectively, demonstrating that both MAPK and FAK play key roles in $\alpha_v\beta_3$-mediated regulation of EGFR activity. A cooperative effect of EGFR and integrins has also been reported in JAK2/STAT3 signaling, which is associated with EMT in cancer [91]. Colomiere *et al.* reported that EGF exposure initiates an EMT-associated increase in N-cadherin and vimentin levels, as well as cell motility in OVCA 433 and SKOV3 cells. Ovarian cancer cells also showed increased activation of JAK2/STAT3 and expression of α_2, α_6, and β_1 integrin subunits when treated with EGF. Blocking integrin subunits α_6 and β_1 significantly inhibited EGF-induced migration, suggesting an interaction between EGFR, $\alpha_6\beta_1$ integrins, and JAK2/STAT3 signaling in ovarian cancer cells that increases EMT and cell motility. The crosstalk between EGFR and β_1 integrin was also studied by Lau *et al.* in the context of invasion and metastasis in ovarian cancer [35]. The authors found that EGF stimulation induces β_1 expression in OVCAR5 and SKOV3 cells, and that blocking the MAPK/ERK pathway inhibited EGF-enhanced β_1 expression. β_1 is downstream of the MAPK/ERK pathway and EGF-induced β_1 expression is mediated by MAPK/ERK signaling. In summary, EGFR plays a key role in multiple cell survival pathways and its overexpression is associated with a poor prognosis in ovarian cancer [84–88]. These studies suggest that EGFR-integrin crosstalk can lead to the potentiation and cooperative stimulation of intracellular pathways that contribute to cell survival and drug resistance.

2.2 The role of FAK, a critical mediator of integrin signaling, in ovarian cancer

As a key player in cell adhesion, motility, and integrin-mediated cell signaling, FAK plays an important role in invasiveness and drug resistance in ovarian cancer. A study by Sood *et al.* reported that FAK is overexpressed in a panel of ovarian cancer cell lines, including SKOV3, EG, and 222, as well as in tissue samples from patients with invasive epithelial ovarian cancer, as compared to normal human ovarian surface epithelial cells and benign ovarian tissue samples [41]. The study showed that the dephosphorylation of FAK by FAK-related nonkinase (FRNK), decreased the invasion and migration of ovarian cancer cells *in vitro*. To evaluate the role of FAK degradation in cisplatin-mediated apoptosis in a cisplatin-sensitive ovarian cancer cell line, Sasaki *et al.* [92] treated OV2008 cells with varying concentrations of cisplatin

(0–10 μM) then analyzed FAK expression in detached cells. Relative to the small number of cells that remained attached following cisplatin treatment, the detached cells expressed low levels of FAK and an increased accumulation of FAK cleavage fragments. Further, morphological investigations on detached cells showed incidence of apoptotic nuclear condensation and fragmentation after 12-hours of incubation with cisplatin. Therefore, the results of this study suggest that cisplatin causes apoptosis in OV2008 cells by caspase-3-mediated FAK cleavage and cell detachment, which can be inhibited by either synthetic or endogenous caspase-3 inhibitors. In another study assessing the mechanism of taxane-based chemotherapeutic agent-mediated apoptosis, Halder *et al.* [93] reported an increase in FAK cleavage and caspase-3 activity in docetaxel-sensitive parental SKOV3 and HeyA8 ovarian cancer cell lines in response to docetaxel treatment. Both FAK cleavage and caspase-3 activity remained unchanged in resistant ovarian cancer cell lines SKOV3-TR and HeyA8-MDR. Furthermore, inhibiting caspase-3 by the caspase blocker, DEVD-fmk, decreased docetaxel-mediated FAK cleavage and apoptosis in parental cells. Similarly, silencing FAK by siRNA transfection increased docetaxel effectiveness in both parental and resistant cell lines.

2.3 Malignant ascites in integrin-mediated invasiveness in ovarian cancer

Malignant ascites, the abnormal accumulation of fluid containing malignant cells in the peritoneum [92, 93], is more frequently associated with advanced-stage ovarian cancer than any other peritoneal malignancy, and represents a barrier to treatment [94, 95]. As shown in **Figure 3**, there are a variety of cellular and acellular factors in malignant ascites that contribute to disease progression, immune evasion, and even chemoresistance in ovarian cancer [92, 96]. Acellular factors

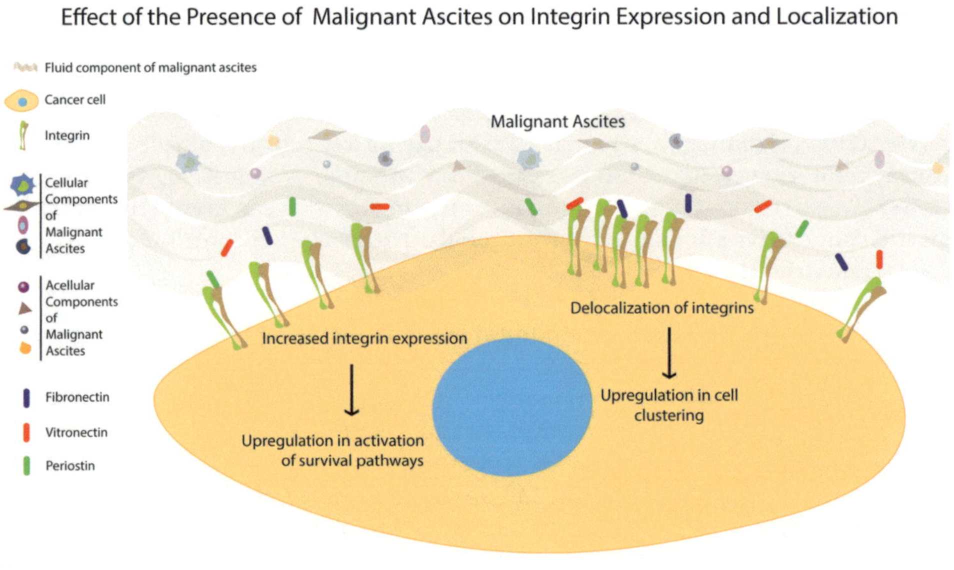

Figure 3.
Malignant ascites has been shown to affect integrin expression and localization. Specifically, cellular and acellular factors in malignant ascites can promote increased integrin expression, leading to the upregulation of integrin-related survival pathways. Factors within malignant ascites can also promote integrin delocalization, which leads to cell clustering.

include integrins, which play a role in the formation of a tumor-promoting microenvironment. Although these adhesion-regulating factors are normally involved in cell differentiation, growth, and migration [11, 97, 98], aberrant integrin signaling frequently observed in cancers can influence cell invasiveness, drug resistance, and metastasis [14].

There are a multitude of integrins that are known to play a role in ovarian cancer. In the normal tumor microenvironment, activation of apoptosis by death receptors plays a key role in immune surveillance against tumor cells [99]. A study performed by Lane *et al.* demonstrated that malignant ascites protects against tumor necrosis factor-related apoptosis-inducing ligand (TRAIL)-induced apoptosis through activation of the PI3K/Akt pathway in ovarian cancer cells. Normally, OVCAR3 and Caov-3 cell lines are sensitive to TRAIL-induced apoptosis and when exposed to TRAIL in the absence of ascites, only about 10% of cells remained viable. In contrast, Caov-3 cells exposed to TRAIL and patient-derived malignant ascites displayed a significant decrease in TRAIL-induced cell death. Similarly, OVCAR3 cells exposed to TRAIL and patient-derived malignant ascites demonstrated significantly increased cell viability compared to those treated only with TRAIL. A follow-up study performed by Lane *et al.* showed that ascites protects against TRAIL-induced apoptosis through $\alpha_v\beta_5$ integrin-mediated FAK and Akt activation [100]. Tumor cells in ascites from ovarian cancer often have higher expression of Akt compared to cells found in benign effusions, which suggests the role of ascites in the activation of the Akt pathway [101]. Akt activation may also occur due to the interactions between ECM proteins and cell surface integrins, integrin-mediated recruitment of FAK, or $\alpha_v\beta_3$ and $\alpha_v\beta_5$ integrin ligation [102–104]. In the study described above by Lane *et al.*, the use of $\alpha_v\beta_3$ and $\alpha_v\beta_5$ integrin-blocking antibodies on Caov-3 cells in the presence of ascites demonstrated a 50% reduction in the protective effect of ascites on TRAIL-induced apoptosis [100]. The addition of $\alpha_v\beta_5$ integrin-blocking antibody also prevented FAK phosphorylation, demonstrating that ascites-induced FAK phosphorylation is $\alpha_v\beta_5$-dependent and that survival factors present in malignant ascites can promote resistance to TRAIL-induced apoptosis through Akt activation in an $\alpha_v\beta_5$-dependent manner [99, 100].

Factors within ascites that engage $\alpha_v\beta_5$ integrins may include vitronectin and periostin, which are ECM proteins secreted by malignant ovarian epithelial cells [100, 103, 105]. Adhesion of ovarian cancer cells to the ECM is controlled by integrin-dependent and independent mechanisms, therefore changes in the ECM composition as well as integrin expression allow for the alteration of cancer cell adhesion and motility [26, 105–108]. Periostin is overexpressed in, and secreted by, epithelial ovarian cancer cells, and as a result, periostin accumulates in the malignant ascites [105, 109]. In a study by Gillan *et al.*, ~95% of ascites samples from ovarian cancer patients contained periostin [105]. Exploring the role of periostin in cell adhesion, Gillan *et al.* found that periostin-coated surfaces supported HOSE and SKOV3 cell attachment in a concentration-dependent manner. SKOV3 cell adhesion was enhanced after adding manganese, which increases the ligand-binding affinity of integrin $\alpha_v\beta_3$; however, adhesion was inhibited by anti-$\alpha_v\beta_3$ and anti-$\alpha_v\beta_5$ antibodies. When examining the role of periostin on ovarian cancer cell motility, Gillan *et al.* further showed that ovarian cancer cells grown on periostin formed less stress fibers and focal adhesion plaques than those grown on vitronectin or fibronectin. Based on these findings, Gillan *et al.* concluded that $\alpha_v\beta_3$ and $\alpha_v\beta_5$ integrin play important roles in periostin-induced effects on cell adhesion and motility, which could promote intraperitoneal dissemination of ovarian cancer.

Similar to periostin, vitronectin and fibronectin are also important in shaping the tumor-promoting microenvironment of malignant ascites. Specifically, fibronectin has been shown to promote cell migration and spheroid formation, anchorage, and disaggregation in ovarian cancer [25, 27, 110, 111], while vitronectin has been found to play key roles in cancer cell adhesion, proliferation, and migration [112–115]. Fibronectin and vitronectin can also enhance metastasis when they are cleaved into smaller fragments by matrix metalloproteinase-2 (MMP-2) [111, 116]. A study by Carduner *et al.* found that, in 14 patient-derived ascites samples, both vitronectin and fibronectin were detected. When cells were grown on patient-derived ascites, their morphology changed to clusters of rounded cells varying in thickness [111]. Purified vitronectin and fibronectin from patient-derived ascites also supported the adhesion and migration of ovarian cancer cells alongside altered integrin organization. Vitronectin-exposed IGROV1, OVCAR3, and SKOV3 cells displayed altered localization and/or organization patterns of α_v and β_1 integrins. In fibronectin-exposed cells, co-localization between β_1 integrin and fibronectin fibrils was observed, suggesting a role for integrins in fibrillation.

Since EMT behavior can also be modulated by ascites in an integrin-dependent manner, Carduner *et al.* examined the EMT status of cells based on cell-cell contact, modification of cell-matrix adhesion, elongation of cell shape, and cell migration [117]. After treatment with ascites, cell shape was altered in IGROV1, SKOV3, and OVCAR3 cells, as cells become clustered, spindle-like, and heterogenous, respectively. Ascites also induced changes in localization and the expression of epithelial and mesenchymal markers that differed by cell line, but were nonetheless associated with an ascites-associated shift towards an intermediate epithelial or mesenchymal phenotype. In IGROV1 and SKOV3 cells, Carduner *et al.* reported that α_v integrins were involved in the observed shift towards a mesenchymal phenotype, since ascites induced the partial delocalization of α_v integrins to favor the formation of IGROV1 aggregates and SKOV3 migration. Overall, this study found that exposure to ascites stimulates integrin trafficking and is associated with a shift towards a mesenchymal phenotype in ovarian cancer cells.

Additional studies have implicated α_v integrins in ovarian cancer progression by promoting an ascites-associated invasive and mesenchymal phenotype. For example, $\alpha_v\beta_6$ integrin has been correlated with increased urokinase plasminogen (uPA) expression, MMP-2 and MMP-9 secretion, and protease-dependent matrix degradation [23, 32]. Increased uPA and MMP-9 expression are associated with a poor prognosis because they contribute to ovarian cancer progression and enhanced metastatic potential [23, 118, 119]. uPA and its receptor (uPAR) are often found at high concentrations in both the tumors and ascitic fluid of advanced-stage ovarian cancer patients [120, 121]. It has been shown that increased uPAR expression in cancer cells is maintained by ERK MAP kinase pathway activity, which is associated with tumor cell growth and proliferation [122–125]. The ERK MAP kinase pathway, a downstream target of the Ras pathway, is often activated upon integrin binding and activation [122, 123]. Since integrins, uPA, and MMPs are all present in malignant ascites, and are associated with a poor prognosis, Ahmed *et al.* examined the role of ascites in regulating integrin-mediated changes in ovarian cancer growth and function [122]. Results showed that, in the presence of ascites, α_6 integrin expression was enhanced in OVHS1, PEO.36, OVCA 433 and HEY cell lines while uPAR expression was only enhanced in invasive OVCA 433 and HEY cell lines. Additionally, while malignant and high-grade tumors displayed epithelial uPAR staining, uPAR expression was absent in normal and benign tumor samples. α_6 integrin staining was also much lower in benign and grade I tumors. Confirming the role of integrins in ovarian cancer cell progression, decreased ascites-induced and basal proliferation were observed in OVHS1 and HEY cell lines incubated with α_6 and β_1 antibodies. Similarly, decreased ascites-induced invasiveness was reported in OVCA 433 and HEY cell lines incubated with α_6, β_1, and uPAR antibodies.

Overall, acellular factors, such as integrins, play critical roles in shaping the ascitic tumor microenvironment of ovarian cancer and contribute to tumor growth, invasion, and metastasis. Since aberrant integrin signaling can increase invasiveness, chemoresistance, and metastasis of cancer cells, understanding the role of ascites and integrin expression in ovarian cancer is crucial for the development of targeted therapies.

3. Integrins in ovarian cancer treatment

The current standard of care for ovarian cancer involves surgical debulking followed by treatment with multiple cycles of platinum- and taxane-based chemotherapy [3]. While this treatment regimen is often effective initially, the rapid development of resistance to these drugs is one of the main challenges in the treatment of ovarian cancer [126]. This has led researchers to seek new treatment strategies, such as targeting cell surface receptors that are overexpressed in cancer and tumor endothelial cells [127, 128]. Since research has shown integrins play an important role in vascular development and mediate the adhesion of disseminated cancer cells [28, 129–133], targeting integrins could be a rational treatment approach in ovarian cancer.

One integrin expressed in proliferating vascular endothelial cells, and some tumor cells, is the $\alpha_v\beta_3$ integrin [134]. In an *in ovo* study from 1994, blocking $\alpha_v\beta_3$ integrin led to the disruption of angiogenesis on a chick chorioallantoic membrane (CAM) and the regression of human melanoma tumors grown on the CAM through the induction of apoptosis in associated angiogenic vascular cells [135]. More recently, the cancer-promoting role of $\alpha_v\beta_3$ integrin was demonstrated *in vitro* in a panel of cancer cell lines, including in ovarian cancer cells [136–141]. These efforts led to preclinical *in vivo* studies using the humanized monoclonal antibody, etaracizumab, to inhibit angiogenesis by blocking $\alpha_v\beta_3$ integrin. The efficacy of etaracizumab in ovarian cancer was explored by Landen *et al.*, who generated orthotopic mouse models of ovarian cancer using three chemotherapy sensitive ovarian cancer cell lines: HeyA8, SKOV3ip1, and A2780ip2 (the “ip” cell lines were generated by injecting parental lines into the peritoneum of a mouse, then harvesting, isolating, and re-culturing the tumor cells) [142]. The authors reported that, after injection of etaracizumab, tumor size was significantly reduced in SKOV3ip1 and HeyA8 models, but not in A2780ip2 models. The underlying reason for this may be poor $\alpha_v\beta_3$ integrin expression in A2780ip2 cells, which was confirmed after flow cytometry and Western Blot analysis. Interestingly, when etaracizumab was combined with paclitaxel, A2780ip2 tumors were reduced in size by 72.8% compared to paclitaxel alone. These findings suggest that while etaracizumab alone did not reduce the size of A2780ip2 tumors, etaracizumab in combination with paclitaxel led to a synergistic reduction in A2780ip2 tumor size. The same synergism was not observed in HeyA8 tumors even though it was effective as a monotherapy, which the authors suggest may be due to the varied roles of the Akt pathway in the three cell lines. Proliferation in HeyA8 cells is driven, in significant part, by the MEK/ERK pathway and not the Akt pathway, while the other two cell lines have constitutive activation of Akt, potentially explaining the observed discrepancies in the efficacy of tumor reduction.

A follow-up study from the same research group assessed the efficacy of combining etaracizumab with the clinically approved VEGF receptor antibody, bevacizumab [143]. Taxane-sensitive (SKOV3ip1 and HeyA8), and -resistant (SKOV3TRip2) tumors were treated with single-agent therapies or with a cocktail of the two antibodies. Additionally, the individual antibodies, or the cocktail, were tested in combination with paclitaxel. In the SKOV3ip1 model, both individual agents as well as the etaracizumab-bevacizumab cocktail reduced tumor size, with the cocktail proving more effective than single agents alone. Furthermore, paclitaxel efficacy was increased in combination with bevacizumab or the cocktail, but not with etaracizumab, in the SKOV3ip1 model. In SKOV3TRip2 cells, bevacizumab or etaracizumab individually sensitized cells to paclitaxel. In HeyA8 cells, while bevacizumab alone significantly reduced tumor weight, neither etaracizumab alone, nor in combination with bevacizumab or paclitaxel, led to significant tumor size reduction, consistent with the findings reported above. Despite the literature supporting the anti-tumor activity of $\alpha_v\beta_3$ inhibition, there is also evidence that $\alpha_v\beta_3$ expression in ovarian cancer cells may inhibit tumor progression and reduce metastasis [144, 145], warranting further investigation into the value of targeting this integrin pair for ovarian cancer treatment.

Another drug that has been evaluated in preclinical and clinical studies for integrin-targeted treatment of ovarian cancer is the humanized $\alpha_5\beta_1$ antibody volociximab. As previously mentioned, α_5 and β_1 integrins have been implicated in ovarian cancer cell adhesion and migration [28, 146]; however, $\alpha_5\beta_1$ integrin is also associated with endothelial cell proliferation and survival [147, 148]. Kim *et al.* [131] blocked $\alpha_5\beta_1$ integrins in human tumors grown on CAMs and found that that $\alpha_5\beta_1$ regulates angiogenesis through the same pathway as $\alpha_v\beta_3$ integrin. Blocking $\alpha_5\beta_1$ integrin using volociximab also proved successful in a cynomolgus monkey model of choroidal neovascularization [147], leading to a phase I clinical trial assessing volociximab in 21 patients with pathologically confirmed solid malignancies in 2008 [149]. After demonstrating safety in phase I trials, volociximab was tested in a single-arm, multi-institutional, phase II study. 14 patients with platinum-resistant, advanced stage epithelial ovarian cancer or primary peritoneal cancer received weekly intravenous volociximab at a dose of 15 mg/kg until progression or unacceptable toxicity. Among the patients whose responses were evaluable, only one patient remained in a stable condition, while the disease of the other 13 patients progressed. Although volociximab did not progress clinically for the treatment of ovarian cancer, the inhibition of neovascularization using the anti-VEGF receptor bevacizumab was approved in 2018 for the treatment of women with advanced (stage III or IV) ovarian cancer in combination with chemotherapy following initial surgical resection [150–152]. Unlike bevacizumab, $\alpha_1\beta_5$ and $\alpha_v\beta_3$ integrins can block multiple growth factor pathways and cause apoptosis of proliferating endothelial cells, thus targeting angiogenesis from multiple routes. Although this strategy seems promising, integrin inhibitor drugs have not been recognized clinically because of inconsistent results and insufficient clinical activity.

Targeting integrins for selective drug delivery is another strategy of interest in the context of ovarian cancer treatment. The arginine-glycine-aspartic acid (RGD) tripeptide motif is found in many ECM proteins including collagen, fibronectin, and vitronectin. Since this motif is recognized by many integrins, chemotherapy agents can be coupled with RGD to deliver them selectively to ovarian cancer cells that overexpress certain integrins. This was shown by Pilkington-Miksa *et al.* who

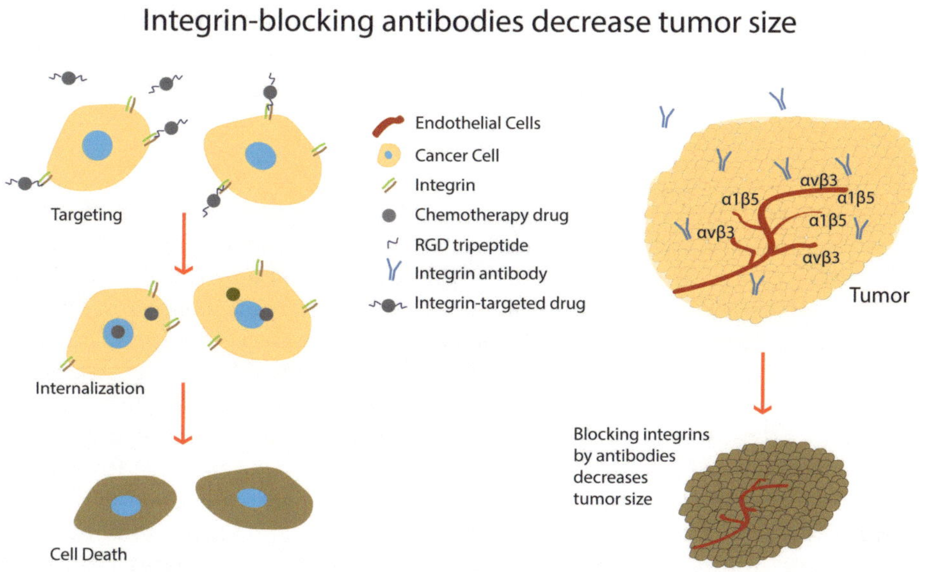

Figure 4.
Integrins as therapeutic targets in ovarian cancer. Integrin-targeted drugs, or anti-integrin antibodies, can be directly toxic to tumor cells that overexpress integrins (left) or can inhibit tumor vasculature (right), thereby decreasing tumor size.

synthesized an $\alpha_v\beta_3$ integrin-binding RGD-paclitaxel conjugate that was more effective than unconjugated paclitaxel at decreasing tumor volume in a xenograft ovarian cancer model [153]. RGD-modified liposomes containing paclitaxel (RGD-SSL-PXT) have also been synthesized and tested in *in vitro* and *in vivo* ovarian cancer cell models [154]. Zhao *et al.* reported that the intracellular uptake of RGD-SSL-PXTs by SKOV3 cells was more than 6-fold higher, relative to non-targeted liposomes, and the tumor inhibition efficacy of RGD-SSL-PXTs was superior to both paclitaxel and non-targeted liposomes containing paclitaxel. In summary, there are a variety of ways that integrins can be targeted to reduce tumor burden in ovarian cancer. Thus far, as demonstrated in **Figure 4**, researchers have explored integrin inhibition in the context of vascular development as well as the selective delivery of RGD-modified cancer therapeutics; however, further research is needed to fully understand the potential value of targeting integrins in ovarian cancer treatment.

4. Targeting integrins for fluorescence imaging and photochemical/ phototthermal treatment in ovarian cancer

Photodynamic therapy (PDT) is a photochemical treatment modality involving the activation of a photosensitive molecule, a photosensitizer (PS), with light of an appropriate wavelength leading to the generation of reactive molecular species at the site of PS localization [155–157]. PSs can be conjugated to proteins or peptides, or formulated in delivery systems, to enhance selectivity or to improve photochemical potency [158–161]. As discussed previously, integrins play an important role in ovarian cancer progression, but targeting integrins for selective drug delivery remains challenging. There are a limited number of studies that focus on integrin targeting in photochemistry-based applications. This section serves as a comprehensive review of the studies that have evaluated the effects of photosensitization on integrins, as well as the studies that target integrins to improve selectivity for fluorescence imaging and PDT of ovarian cancer. One photothermal therapy (PTT) study is also discussed at the end of this section to cover light-based practices that target integrins in ovarian cancer [162].

The effect of PDT on integrin expression and reorganization has been studied in the context of ovarian cancer by Runnels *et al.* [163]. In this study, OVCAR3 cells were maintained in monolayer or injected intraperitoneally into nude mice. *In vitro* and *in vivo* PDT treatments were carried out using a 690 nm argon ion pumped dye laser at 0.5 J/cm^2 energy density following a 3-hour incubation of the cells with 0.092 μmol/L benzoporphyrin derivative monoacid (BPD). Subsequently, the cells were harvested and re-seeded on surfaces coated with ECM proteins: collagen IV, fibronectin, laminin, and vitronectin. Low-dose PDT (~ 85% cell survival) was shown to decrease the adhesion of OVCAR3 cells to collagen IV, fibronectin, laminin, and vitronectin-coated substrates *in vitro* and *in vivo*. The authors further reported that the binding of OVCAR3 cells to collagen IV and laminin, but not fibronectin, was inhibited by the presence of an anti-β1 antibody, suggesting that the β1 subunit plays a role in the adhesion of OVCAR3 cells to select ECM proteins. It was also noted that BPD localized in and around mitochondria and caused intracellular damage upon irradiation, mainly mediated by singlet oxygen rather than other reactive molecular species. In this study, BPD-PDT-mediated photodamage was shown to impact integrin function and the integrity of focal adhesion plaques.

A limited number of studies have explored integrins as targets for selective delivery of imaging agents and PSs. In a recent study, Li and colleagues linked an RGD-peptide and IRDye 700 DX (IR700) to human serum albumin [164]. Compared to the untargeted nanoconjugate, cell delivery of the targeted nanoconjugate (cRGD-PEG-HSA-IR700) increased by 121-fold in $\alpha_v\beta_3$-expressing TOV21G cells. Cells were also treated using a 660 nm LED light source at an irradiance of 3.5 mW/cm^2 for 20 minutes [a fluence of 4.2 J/cm^2, not specified in the report]. PDT effectively killed the $\alpha_v\beta_3$-expressing TOV21G cells but did not affect $\alpha_v\beta_3$-negative NIH/3 T3 cells. The nanoconjugates were also tested on spheroids of SKOV3 cells grown in ultra-low attachment wells. Confocal microscopy images and live/dead staining assays revealed that cRGD-PEG-HSA-IR700 successfully penetrated the spheroids, generated cell killing, and caused long-term tumor suppression. An RGD peptide with EtNBS as the PS and a 5 kDa polyethylene glycol (PEG) chain has also been explored in the context of ovarian cancer [165]. Using this construct, cellular uptake was increased in genetically modified, α_5 integrin-overexpressing OVCAR5 cells relative to wild-type OVCAR5 cells. PEGylated constructs aggregated less and generated more reactive molecular species compared to their non-PEGylated analogs. Dai *et al.* synthesized a compound called TTB, which exhibits aggregation-induced near infrared (NIR) fluorescence and generates reactive oxygen species when excited by white light [166]. TTB was integrated into an amphiphilic polymer 1,2-distearoyl-sn-glycero-3-phosphoethanolamine-N-[maleimide(polyethylene glycol)-2000] (MPD) and conjugated with RGD peptide to target $\alpha_v\beta_3$ integrins. Efficacy of the construct for PDT and fluorescence imaging was evaluated *in vitro* and in animal models of prostate, cervical, and ovarian cancer. The integrin-targeted construct was shown to selectively accumulate in tumors, leading to cancer cell death *in vitro* and reduction of tumor size in tumor-bearing mice, compared to controls.

Fluorescence imaging of cancer relies on the selective accumulation of fluorescent agents in cancer cells. $\alpha_v\beta_3$ integrins are the most common targets in integrin-targeted fluorescent imaging studies. For instance, the fluorescent probe squaraine was covalently attached to one (monovalent) and two (divalent) cyclic RGD peptides by Shaw and colleagues to target ovarian cancer cells that overexpress $\alpha_v\beta_3$ integrins [167]. Uptake of the divalent probe in OVCAR4 cells was 2.2-fold higher than the monovalent probe, based on fluorescence imaging. Consistently, tumors grown in nude mice and imaged with the divalent probe were almost three times more fluorescent compared to tumors given the monovalent probe, and six times more fluorescent than tumors that received non-conjugated squaraine. To explore the potential of integrin-targeted, fluorescence-guided resection in ovarian cancer, Alvero *et al.* created a PLGA-PEG nanoparticle to target $\alpha_v\beta_3$ integrins in OCSC1-F2 ovarian cancer cells using an RGD peptide and three different fluorescent dyes: DIR, C6, and ICG [168]. The resulting conjugates enabled the investigators to visualize both the tumor-associated vasculature and intraperitoneal ovarian cancer micrometastases as small as 100 μm in a xenograft model. These studies demonstrate the potential of using $\alpha_v\beta_3$-targeted agents for fluorescence guided resection in ovarian cancer. An additional important consideration for this approach is the accuracy of tumor detection. This concern was addressed in a study by Harlaar *et al.*, who found that the diagnostic accuracy of an $\alpha_v\beta_3$-targeted agent in combination with an NIR fluorescence intra-operative imaging system was 96.5%, with a sensitivity of 95% and a specificity of 88% [169].

In comparison to RGD peptides that have been relatively widely used to target integrins, less commonly used peptides, such as "OA02", have been synthesized to bind an α_3 integrin subunit [170]. An *in vivo* study by Aina *et al.* used nude mice bearing ES-2 tumors to evaluate three different forms of this peptide: OA02-biotin-Cy5.5, OA02-Cy5.5, and OA02-AlexaFluo 680. Results showed that OA02-Cy5.5 and OA02-AlexaFluo 680 exhibited fast and specific tumor uptake that sustained a fluorescence signal for approximately 70 minutes. Although the cellular uptake of OA02-biotin-Cy5.5 was slower than other peptide variants, the duration of the fluorescence signal was 24 hours. To confirm that α_3 integrins were mediating the binding of OA02 peptides to ES-2 tumors, mice were injected with an anti-α_3 monoclonal antibody, which blocked binding of the peptides to the tumors.

The value of targeting integrins has also been explored in the context of PTT, which involves the interaction of electromagnetic radiation (typically NIR light) with a photothermal agent to generate heat, leading to tissue hyperthermia. In a study by Zhou *et al.*, the selectivity of silica-coated gold nanorods for ovarian cancer cells increased using hyaluronic acid and an RGD peptide that bind to CD44 and $\alpha_v\beta_3$ integrin, respectively [171]. The targeted nanoparticle showed high selectivity for SKOV3 cells but not for non-cancerous HOSEpiC cells. The nanorods were also loaded with doxorubicin (DOX) to increase cytotoxicity. PTT using the dual-targeted, DOX-loaded gold nanorods, and irradiation with an 808 nm laser at a high-power density (2 W/cm^2), exhibited the highest cytotoxicity to SKOV3 cells among all experimental groups. Subsequent experiments have revealed that the release of DOX is pH-sensitive and triggered by NIR irradiation. DOX release may be influenced by hyaluronidase-mediated degradation of hyaluronic acid in low pH environments, and the disruption of the interaction between DOX and silica, respectively. An overview of photochemistry-based studies that focus on modulating or targeting integrins in the context of ovarian cancer is presented in **Figure 5**.

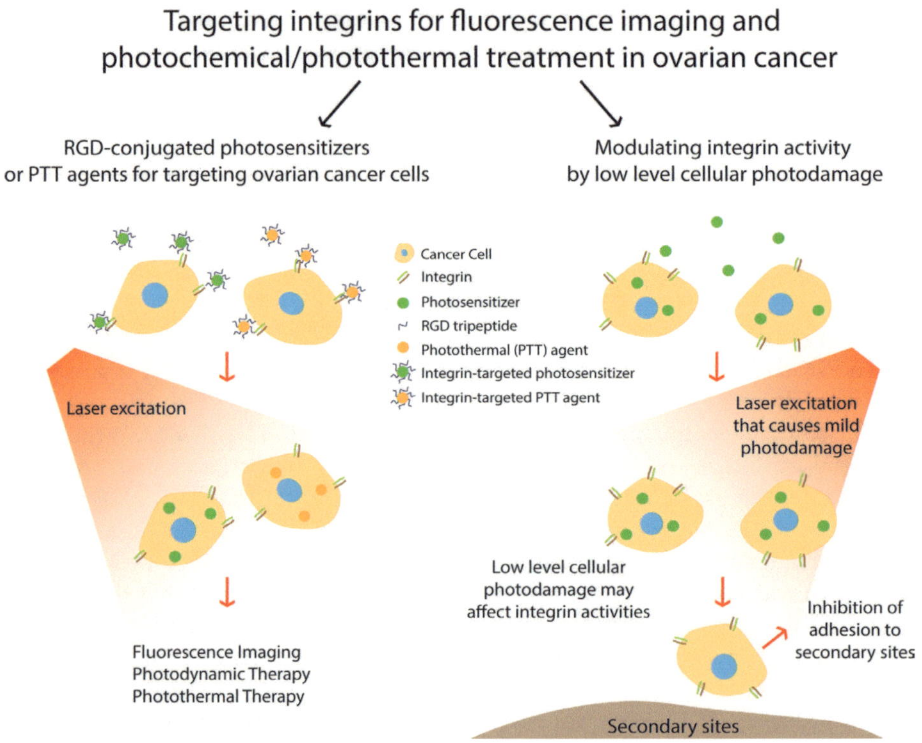

Figure 5.
Integrins as targets for fluorescence imaging and photochemical or photothermal treatment in ovarian cancer. Current research focuses on using RGD tripeptide-conjugated PS or PTT agents to target ovarian cancer cells that overexpress integrins (left), or to modulate integrin activity and inhibit cancer cell adhesion to secondary sites by low level cellular photodamage (right).

In summary, targeting integrins is a promising strategy for both anti-cancer PDT and fluorescence imaging. Since most PSs also have fluorescent properties, novel nanocarriers with integrin-targeting molecules can be used in theranostic applications and in real-time image-guided PDT of ovarian cancer. The potential of integrin-targeted PDT warrants further evaluation.

5. Conclusion

Integrins are key players in cell adhesion and cell-ECM interactions that mediate important cell functions, such as survival, differentiation, and migration. In cancer, the aberrant expression, or reorganization, of integrins are associated with critical steps in tumor progression. Studies assessing the role of integrins in the context of ovarian cancer revealed that integrins are involved in ovarian cancer cell survival, migration, adhesion, and invasion of secondary sites. Despite this, integrin-targeted drugs for the treatment of ovarian cancer have displayed limited clinical success and have largely been evaluated in pre-clinical studies. Targeting integrins that are overexpressed in cancer cells for imaging or treatment purposes, using photochemical strategies, is a promising research area. Integrin function can be manipulated by

PDT or a PS can be conjugated to target ovarian cancer cells that overexpress certain integrins for fluorescence imaging or toxicity via photodamage. Due to the role that integrins play during critical steps in ovarian cancer progression, integrin targeting may be promising for inhibition of tumor vasculature, drug delivery and photochemistry-based applications in ovarian cancer.

Acknowledgements

This work was supported, in part, by the National Institutes of Health (NIH), a pre-doctoral traineeship from (National Research Service Award T32 ES007126 to BPR) from National Institute of Environmental Health Sciences (NIEHS), an NIH T32 award to the Certificate in Translational Medicine Program at UNC-Chapel Hill: grant number GM122741 (to BPR), as well as funding from the NC Translational and Clinical Sciences Institute (NC TraCS) at UNC-Chapel Hill supported by the National Center for Advancing Translational Sciences (NCATS), NIH through Grant Award Number UL1TR002489 (to WJP and IR), the Center for Environmental Health and Susceptibility (CEHS) at UNC-Chapel Hill supported by the NIEHS through Grant Award Number P30ES010126 (to IR), and UNC-NC State Joint Department of Biomedical Engineering Startup Funds (to WJP and IR). The content is solely the responsibility of the authors and does not necessarily represent the official views of the National Institutes of Health.

Author details

Mustafa Kemal Ruhi[1,2], Brittany P. Rickard[1,3], William J. Polacheck[1,4,5] and Imran Rizvi[1,3,5]*

1 Joint Department of Biomedical Engineering, University of North Carolina at Chapel Hill, Chapel Hill, NC, and North Carolina State University, Raleigh, NC, USA

2 Institute of Biomedical Engineering, Boğaziçi University, Istanbul, Turkey

3 Curriculum in Toxicology and Environmental Medicine, School of Medicine, University of North Carolina at Chapel Hill, Chapel Hill, NC, USA

4 Department of Cell Biology and Physiology, University of North Carolina School of Medicine, Chapel Hill, NC, USA

5 Lineberger Comprehensive Cancer Center, University of North Carolina School of Medicine, Chapel Hill, NC, USA

*Address all correspondence to: imran.rizvi@unc.edu

References

[1] Siegel RL, Miller KD, Jemal A. Cancer statistics, 2020. CA: A Cancer Journal for Clinicians. 2020;**70**(1):7-30

[2] Torre LA, Trabert B, DeSantis CE, Miller KD, Samimi G, Runowicz CD, et al. Ovarian cancer statistics, 2018. CA: A Cancer Journal for Clinicians. 2018;**68**(4):284-296

[3] Lengyel E. Ovarian cancer development and metastasis. The American Journal of Pathology. 2010;**177**(3):1053-1064

[4] Tan DS, Agarwal R, Kaye SB. Mechanisms of transcoelomic metastasis in ovarian cancer. The Lancet Oncology. 2006;**7**(11):925-934

[5] Dhaliwal D, Shepherd TG. Molecular and cellular mechanisms controlling integrin-mediated cell adhesion and tumor progression in ovarian cancer metastasis: A review. Clinical & Experimental Metastasis. 2022;**39**(2):291-301

[6] Hynes RO. Integrins: A family of cell surface receptors. Cell. 1987;**48**(4):549-554

[7] Hynes RO. Integrins: Bidirectional, allosteric signaling machines. Cell. 2002;**110**(6):673-687

[8] Schwartz MA, Schaller MD, Ginsberg MH. Integrins: Emerging paradigms of signal transduction. Annual Review of Cell and Developmental Biology. 1995;**11**:549-599

[9] Humphries JD, Chastney MR, Askari JA, Humphries MJ. Signal transduction via integrin adhesion complexes. Current Opinion in Cell Biology. 2019;**56**:14-21

[10] Geiger B, Spatz JP, Bershadsky AD. Environmental sensing through focal adhesions. Nature Reviews. Molecular Cell Biology. 2009;**10**(1):21-33

[11] Schoenwaelder SM, Burridge K. Bidirectional signaling between the cytoskeleton and integrins. Current Opinion in Cell Biology. 1999;**11**(2): 274-286

[12] Moore SW, Roca-Cusachs P, Sheetz MP. Stretchy proteins on stretchy substrates: The important elements of integrin-mediated rigidity sensing. Developmental Cell. 2010;**19**(2): 194-206

[13] Ginsberg MH, Du X, Plow EF. Inside-out integrin signalling. Current Opinion in Cell Biology. 1992;**4**(5):766-771

[14] Hamidi H, Ivaska J. Every step of the way: Integrins in cancer progression and metastasis. Nature Reviews Cancer. 2018;**18**(9):533-548

[15] Lu P, Weaver VM, Werb Z. The extracellular matrix: A dynamic niche in cancer progression. The Journal of Cell Biology. 2012;**196**(4):395-406

[16] Pickup MW, Mouw JK, Weaver VM. The extracellular matrix modulates the hallmarks of cancer. EMBO Reports. 2014;**15**(12):1243-1253

[17] Ghosh S, Wu Y, Stack MS. Ovarian cancer-associated proteinases. Cancer Treatment and Research. 2002;**107**:331-351

[18] Symowicz J, Adley BP, Gleason KJ, Johnson JJ, Ghosh S, Fishman DA, et al. Engagement of collagen-binding integrins promotes matrix metalloproteinase-9-dependent E-cadherin ectodomain shedding

in ovarian carcinoma cells. Cancer Research. 2007;**67**(5):2030-2039

[19] Lochter A, Galosy S, Muschler J, Freedman N, Werb Z, Bissell MJ. Matrix metalloproteinase stromelysin-1 triggers a cascade of molecular alterations that leads to stable epithelial-to-mesenchymal conversion and a premalignant phenotype in mammary epithelial cells. The Journal of Cell Biology. 1997;**139**(7):1861-1872

[20] Dwivedi DJ, Pino G, Banh A, Nathu Z, Howchin D, Margetts P, et al. Matrix metalloproteinase inhibitors suppress transforming growth factor-beta-induced subcapsular cataract formation. The American Journal of Pathology. 2006;**168**(1):69-79

[21] Niu J, Gu X, Turton J, Meldrum C, Howard EW, Agrez M. Integrin-mediated signalling of gelatinase B secretion in colon cancer cells. Biochemical and Biophysical Research Communications. 1998;**249**(1):287-291

[22] Thomas GJ, Poomsawat S, Lewis MP, Hart IR, Speight PM, Marshall JF. Alpha v beta 6 integrin upregulates matrix metalloproteinase 9 and promotes migration of normal oral keratinocytes. The Journal of Investigative Dermatology. 2001;**116**(6):898-904

[23] Ahmed N, Riley C, Rice GE, Quinn MA, Baker MS. Alpha(v)beta(6) integrin-a marker for the malignant potential of epithelial ovarian cancer. The Journal of Histochemistry and Cytochemistry: Official Journal of the Histochemistry Society. 2002;**50**(10):1371-1380

[24] Slack-Davis JK, Atkins KA, Harrer C, Hershey ED, Conaway M. Vascular cell adhesion molecule-1 is a regulator of ovarian cancer peritoneal metastasis. Cancer Research. 2009;**69**(4):1469-1476

[25] Casey RC, Burleson KM, Skubitz KM, Pambuccian SE, Oegema TR, Ruff LE, et al. B1-Integrins regulate the formation and adhesion of ovarian carcinoma multicellular spheroids. American Journal of Pathology. 2001;**159**(6): 2071-2080

[26] Strobel T, Cannistra SA. Beta1-integrins partly mediate binding of ovarian cancer cells to peritoneal mesothelium in vitro. Gynecologic Oncology. 1999;**73**(3):362-367

[27] Burleson KM, Casey RC, Skubitz KM, Pambuccian SE, Oegema TR Jr, Skubitz AP. Ovarian carcinoma ascites spheroids adhere to extracellular matrix components and mesothelial cell monolayers. Gynecologic Oncology. 2004;**93**(1):170-181

[28] Sawada K, Mitra AK, Radjabi AR, Bhaskar V, Kistner EO, Tretiakova M, et al. Loss of E-cadherin promotes ovarian cancer metastasis via alpha 5-integrin, which is a therapeutic target. Cancer Research. 2008;**68**(7):2329-2339

[29] Kong DH, Kim YK, Kim MR, Jang JH, Lee S. Emerging roles of vascular cell adhesion Molecule-1 (VCAM-1) in immunological disorders and cancer. International Journal of Molecular Sciences. 2018;**19**(4):1057

[30] Zheng W, Ge D, Meng G. Reversing microtubule-directed chemotherapeutic drug resistance by co-delivering alpha2beta1 inhibitor and paclitaxel with nanoparticles in ovarian cancer. Cell Biology International. 2020;**44**(2):610-620

[31] Ahmed N, Niu J, Dorahy DJ, Gu X, Andrews S, Meldrum CJ, et al. Direct integrin alphavbeta6-ERK binding: Implications for tumour growth. Oncogene. 2002;**21**(9):1370-1380

[32] Ahmed N, Pansino F, Baker M, Rice G, Quinn M. Association between alphavbeta6 integrin expression, elevated p42/44 kDa MAPK, and plasminogen-dependent matrix degradation in ovarian cancer. Journal of Cellular Biochemistry. 2002;**84**(4):675-686

[33] Crampton SP, Wu B, Park EJ, Kim JH, Solomon C, Waterman ML, et al. Integration of the beta-catenin-dependent Wnt pathway with integrin signaling through the adaptor molecule Grb2. PLoS One. 2009;**4**(11):e7841

[34] Lossner D, Abou-Ajram C, Benge A, Reuning U. Integrin alphavbeta3 mediates upregulation of epidermal growth-factor receptor expression and activity in human ovarian cancer cells. The International Journal of Biochemistry & Cell Biology. 2008;**40**(12):2746-2761

[35] Lau MT, So WK, Leung PC. Integrin beta1 mediates epithelial growth factor-induced invasion in human ovarian cancer cells. Cancer Letters. 2012;**320**(2):198-204

[36] Mitra SK, Schlaepfer DD. Integrin-regulated FAK-Src signaling in normal and cancer cells. Current Opinion in Cell Biology. 2006;**18**(5):516-523

[37] Fonar Y, Frank D. FAK and WNT signaling: The meeting of two pathways in cancer and development. Anti-Cancer Agents in Medicinal Chemistry. 2011;**11**(7):600-606

[38] Yee KL, Weaver VM, Hammer DA. Integrin-mediated signalling through the MAP-kinase pathway. IET Systems Biology. 2008;**2**(1):8-15

[39] Chen Q, Lin TH, Der CJ, Juliano RL. Integrin-mediated activation of MEK and mitogen-activated protein kinase is independent of Ras [corrected]. The Journal of Biological Chemistry. 1996;**271**(30):18122-18127

[40] Totaro A, Panciera T, Piccolo S. YAP/TAZ upstream signals and downstream responses. Nature Cell Biology. 2018;**20**(8):888-899

[41] Sood AK, Coffin JE, Schneider GB, Fletcher MS, DeYoung BR, Gruman LM, et al. Biological significance of focal adhesion kinase in ovarian cancer: Role in migration and invasion. The American Journal of Pathology. 2004;**165**(4):1087-1095

[42] Kang Y, Hu W, Ivan C, Dalton HJ, Miyake T, Pecot CV, et al. Role of focal adhesion kinase in regulating YB-1-mediated paclitaxel resistance in ovarian cancer. Journal of the National Cancer Institute. 2013;**105**(19):1485-1495

[43] Xu B, Lefringhouse J, Liu Z, West D, Baldwin LA, Ou C, et al. Inhibition of the integrin/FAK signaling axis and c-Myc synergistically disrupts ovarian cancer malignancy. Oncogene. 2017;**6**(1):e295

[44] Fresno Vara JA, Casado E, de Castro J, Cejas P, Belda-Iniesta C, Gonzalez-Baron M. PI3K/Akt signalling pathway and cancer. Cancer Treatment Reviews. 2004;**30**(2):193-204

[45] Osaki M, Oshimura M, Ito H. PI3K-Akt pathway: Its functions and alterations in human cancer. Apoptosis. 2004;**9**(6):667-676

[46] McCubrey JA, Steelman LS, Chappell WH, Abrams SL, Wong EW, Chang F, et al. Roles of the Raf/MEK/ERK pathway in cell growth, malignant transformation and drug resistance. Biochimica et Biophysica Acta. 2007;**1773**(8):1263-1284

[47] Dhillon AS, Hagan S, Rath O, Kolch W. MAP kinase signalling

pathways in cancer. Oncogene. 2007;**26**(22):3279-3290

[48] Kim EK, Choi EJ. Pathological roles of MAPK signaling pathways in human diseases. Biochimica et Biophysica Acta. 2010;**1802**(4):396-405

[49] Assoian RK, Schwartz MA. Coordinate signaling by integrins and receptor tyrosine kinases in the regulation of G1 phase cell-cycle progression. Current Opinion in Genetics & Development. 2001;**11**(1):48-53

[50] Giancotti FG. Integrin signaling: Specificity and control of cell survival and cell cycle progression. Current Opinion in Cell Biology. 1997;**9**(5):691-700

[51] Salaroglio IC, Mungo E, Gazzano E, Kopecka J, Riganti C. ERK is a pivotal player of chemo-immune-resistance in cancer. International Journal of Molecular Sciences. 2019;**20**(10):2505

[52] Shinderman-Maman E, Cohen K, Weingarten C, Nabriski D, Twito O, Baraf L, et al. The thyroid hormone-alphavbeta3 integrin axis in ovarian cancer: Regulation of gene transcription and MAPK-dependent proliferation. Oncogene. 2016;**35**(15):1977-1987

[53] MacKeigan JP, Collins TS, Ting JP. MEK inhibition enhances paclitaxel-induced tumor apoptosis. The Journal of Biological Chemistry. 2000;**275**(50):38953-38956

[54] Liu S, Zha J, Lei M. Inhibiting ERK/Mnk/eIF4E broadly sensitizes ovarian cancer response to chemotherapy. Clinical & Translational Oncology. 2018;**20**(3):374-381

[55] Logan CY, Nusse R. The Wnt signaling pathway in development and disease. Annual Review of Cell and Developmental Biology. 2004;**20**:781-810

[56] Steinhart Z, Angers S. Wnt signaling in development and tissue homeostasis. Development. 2018;**145**(11):dev.146589

[57] Montcouquiol M, Crenshaw EB 3rd, Kelley MW. Noncanonical Wnt signaling and neural polarity. Annual Review of Neuroscience. 2006;**29**:363-386

[58] Polakis P. Wnt signaling and cancer. Genes & Development. 2000;**14**(15):1837-1851

[59] Arend RC, Londono-Joshi AI, Straughn JM Jr, Buchsbaum DJ. The Wnt/beta-catenin pathway in ovarian cancer: A review. Gynecologic Oncology. 2013;**131**(3):772-779

[60] Chikazawa N, Tanaka H, Tasaka T, Nakamura M, Tanaka M, Onishi H, et al. Inhibition of Wnt signaling pathway decreases chemotherapy-resistant side-population colon cancer cells. Anticancer Research. 2010;**30**(6):2041-2048

[61] Cui J, Jiang W, Wang S, Wang L, Xie K. Role of Wnt/beta-catenin signaling in drug resistance of pancreatic cancer. Current Pharmaceutical Design. 2012;**18**(17):2464-2471

[62] Nagaraj AB, Joseph P, Kovalenko O, Singh S, Armstrong A, Redline R, et al. Critical role of Wnt/beta-catenin signaling in driving epithelial ovarian cancer platinum resistance. Oncotarget. 2015;**6**(27):23720-23734

[63] Zhang Z, Cheng L, Li J, Farah E, Atallah NM, Pascuzzi PE, et al. Inhibition of the Wnt/beta-catenin pathway overcomes resistance to enzalutamide in castration-resistant prostate cancer. Cancer Research. 2018;**78**(12):3147-3162

[64] Viscarra T, Buchegger K, Jofre I, Riquelme I, Zanella L, Abanto M, et al. Functional and transcriptomic characterization of carboplatin-resistant

A2780 ovarian cancer cell line. Biological Research. 2019;**52**(1):13

[65] Wu YH, Chang TH, Huang YF, Huang HD, Chou CY. COL11A1 promotes tumor progression and predicts poor clinical outcome in ovarian cancer. Oncogene. 2014;**33**(26):3432-3440

[66] Burkhalter RJ, Symowicz J, Hudson LG, Gottardi CJ, Stack MS. Integrin regulation of beta-catenin signaling in ovarian carcinoma. The Journal of Biological Chemistry. 2011;**286**(26):23467-23475

[67] Dupont S, Morsut L, Aragona M, Enzo E, Giulitti S, Cordenonsi M, et al. Role of YAP/TAZ in mechanotransduction. Nature. 2011;**474**(7350):179-183

[68] Piccolo S, Dupont S, Cordenonsi M. The biology of YAP/TAZ: Hippo signaling and beyond. Physiological Reviews. 2014;**94**(4):1287-1312

[69] Harvey KF, Zhang X, Thomas DM. The hippo pathway and human cancer. Nature Reviews. Cancer. 2013;**13**(4): 246-257

[70] Varelas X. The hippo pathway effectors TAZ and YAP in development, homeostasis and disease. Development. 2014;**141**(8):1614-1626

[71] Azzolin L, Panciera T, Soligo S, Enzo E, Bicciato S, Dupont S, et al. YAP/TAZ incorporation in the beta-catenin destruction complex orchestrates the Wnt response. Cell. 2014;**158**(1):157-170

[72] Rausch V, Hansen CG. The hippo pathway, YAP/TAZ, and the plasma membrane. Trends in Cell Biology. 2020;**30**(1):32-48

[73] Hall CA, Wang R, Miao J, Oliva E, Shen X, Wheeler T, et al. Hippo pathway effector Yap is an ovarian cancer oncogene. Cancer Research. 2010;**70**(21):8517-8525

[74] Zhang X, George J, Deb S, Degoutin JL, Takano EA, Fox SB, et al. The hippo pathway transcriptional co-activator, YAP, is an ovarian cancer oncogene. Oncogene. 2011;**30**(25):2810-2822

[75] Wei X, Jia Y, Lou H, Ma J, Huang Q, Meng Y, et al. Targeting YAP suppresses ovarian cancer progression through regulation of the PI3K/Akt/mTOR pathway. Oncology Reports. 2019;**42**(6):2768-2776

[76] Xia Y, Chang T, Wang Y, Liu Y, Li W, Li M, et al. YAP promotes ovarian cancer cell tumorigenesis and is indicative of a poor prognosis for ovarian cancer patients. PLoS One. 2014;**9**(3):e91770

[77] Xiao L, Shi XY, Zhang Y, Zhu Y, Zhu L, Tian W, et al. YAP induces cisplatin resistance through activation of autophagy in human ovarian carcinoma cells. Oncotargets and Therapy. 2016;**9**:1105-1114

[78] Jeong GO, Shin SH, Seo EJ, Kwon YW, Heo SC, Kim KH, et al. TAZ mediates lysophosphatidic acid-induced migration and proliferation of epithelial ovarian cancer cells. Cellular Physiology and Biochemistry. 2013;**32**(2):253-263

[79] Chen G, Xie J, Huang P, Yang Z. Overexpression of TAZ promotes cell proliferation, migration and epithelial-mesenchymal transition in ovarian cancer. Oncology Letters. 2016;**12**(3):1821-1825

[80] Li G, Hu X, Nie P, Mang D, Jiao S, Zhang S, et al. Lipid-raft-targeted molecular self-assembly inactivates YAP to treat ovarian cancer. Nano Letters. 2021;**21**(1):747-755

[81] Tan G, Cao X, Dai Q, Zhang B, Huang J, Xiong S, et al. A novel role for microRNA-129-5p in inhibiting ovarian cancer cell proliferation and survival via direct suppression of transcriptional co-activators YAP and TAZ. Oncotarget. 2015;**6**(11):8676-8686

[82] Yang WH, Huang Z, Wu J, Ding CC, Murphy SK, Chi JT. A TAZ-ANGPTL4-NOX2 Axis regulates Ferroptotic cell death and Chemoresistance in epithelial ovarian cancer. Molecular Cancer Research. 2020;**18**(1):79-90

[83] Wee P, Wang Z. Epidermal growth factor receptor cell proliferation signaling pathways. Cancers (Basel). 2017;**9**(5):52

[84] Jorissen RN, Walker F, Pouliot N, Garrett TP, Ward CW, Burgess AW. Epidermal growth factor receptor: Mechanisms of activation and signalling. Experimental Cell Research. 2003;**284**(1):31-53

[85] Psyrri A, Kassar M, Yu Z, Bamias A, Weinberger PM, Markakis S, et al. Effect of epidermal growth factor receptor expression level on survival in patients with epithelial ovarian cancer. Clinical Cancer Research. 2005;**11**(24 Pt 1): 8637-8643

[86] Mendelsohn J, Baselga J. Status of epidermal growth factor receptor antagonists in the biology and treatment of cancer. Journal of Clinical Oncology. 2003;**21**(14):2787-2799

[87] Mehner C, Oberg AL, Goergen KM, Kalli KR, Maurer MJ, Nassar A, et al. EGFR as a prognostic biomarker and therapeutic target in ovarian cancer: Evaluation of patient cohort and literature review. Genes & Cancer. 2017;**8**(5-6):589-599

[88] Siwak DR, Carey M, Hennessy BT, Nguyen CT, McGahren Murray MJ, Nolden L, et al. Targeting the epidermal growth factor receptor in epithelial ovarian cancer: Current knowledge and future challenges. Journal of Oncology. 2010;**2010**:568938

[89] Cabodi S, Moro L, Bergatto E, Boeri Erba E, Di Stefano P, Turco E, et al. Integrin regulation of epidermal growth factor (EGF) receptor and of EGF-dependent responses. Biochemical Society Transactions. 2004;**32**(Pt3):438-442

[90] Moro L, Venturino M, Bozzo C, Silengo L, Altruda F, Beguinot L, et al. Integrins induce activation of EGF receptor: Role in MAP kinase induction and adhesion-dependent cell survival. The EMBO Journal. 1998;**17**(22):6622-6632

[91] Colomiere M, Findlay J, Ackland L, Ahmed N. Epidermal growth factor-induced ovarian carcinoma cell migration is associated with JAK2/STAT3 signals and changes in the abundance and localization of alpha6beta1 integrin. The International Journal of Biochemistry & Cell Biology. 2009;**41**(5):1034-1045

[92] Ahmed N, Stenvers KL. Getting to know ovarian cancer ascites: Opportunities for targeted therapy-based translational research. Frontiers in Oncology. 2013;**3**(September):256

[93] Sangisetty SL, Miner TJ. Malignant ascites: A review of prognostic factors, pathophysiology and therapeutic measures. World Journal of Gastrointestinal Surgery. 2012;**4**(4):87-95

[94] Kipps E, Tan DSPP, Kaye SB. Meeting the challenge of ascites in ovarian cancer: New avenues for therapy and research. Nature Reviews Cancer. 2013;**13**(4):273-282

[95] Parsons SL, Lang MW, Steele RJC. Malignant ascites: A 2-year review

from a teaching hospital. European Journal of Surgical Oncology (EJSO). 1996;**22**(3):237-239

[96] Kim S, Kim B, Song YS. Ascites modulates cancer cell behavior, contributing to tumor heterogeneity in ovarian cancer. Cancer Science. 2016;**107**(9):1173-1178

[97] Ginsberg MH, Partridge A, Shattil SJ. Integrin regulation. Current Opinion in Cell Biology. 2005;**17**(5 SPEC. ISS):509-516

[98] Harburger DS, Calderwood DA. Integrin signalling at a glance. Journal of Cell Science. 2009;**122**(9):159-163

[99] Lane D, Robert V, Grondin R, Rancourt C, Piché A. Malignant ascites protect against TRAIL-induced apoptosis by activating the PI3K/Akt pathway in human ovarian carcinoma cells. International journal of cancer. 2007;**121**(6):1227-1237

[100] Lane D, Goncharenko-Khaider N, Rancourt C, Piche A. Ovarian cancer ascites protects from TRAIL-induced cell death through alphavbeta5 integrin-mediated focal adhesion kinase and Akt activation. Oncogene. 2010;**29**(24):3519-3531

[101] Davidson B, Espina V, Steinberg SM, Flørenes VA, Liotta LA, Kristensen GB, et al. Proteomic analysis of malignant ovarian cancer effusions as a tool for biologic and prognostic profiling. Clinical Cancer Research: An Official Journal of the American Association for Cancer Research. 2006;**12**(3 Pt 1):791-799

[102] Hynes RO. Integrins: Versatility, modulation, and signaling in cell adhesion. Cell. 1992;**69**(1):11-25

[103] Stupack DG, Cheresh DA. Get a ligand, get a life: Integrins, signaling and cell survival. Journal of Cell Science. 2002;**115**(Pt 19):3729-3738

[104] Cruet-Hennequart S, Maubant S, Luis J, Gauduchon P, Staedel C, Dedhar S. Alpha(v) integrins regulate cell proliferation through integrin-linked kinase (ILK) in ovarian cancer cells. Oncogene. 2003;**22**(11):1688-1702

[105] Gillan L, Matei D, Fishman DA, Gerbin CS, Karlan BY, Chang DD. Periostin secreted by epithelial ovarian carcinoma is a ligand for αVβ3 and αVβ5 integrins and promotes cell motility. Cancer Research. 2002;**62**(18):5358-5364

[106] Carreiras F, Cruet S, Staedel C, Sichel F, Gauduchon P. Human ovarian adenocarcinoma cells synthesize vitronectin and use it to organize their adhesion. Gynecologic Oncology. 1999;**72**(3):312-322

[107] Cruet S, Salamanca C, Mitchell GWE, Auersperg N. αvβ3 and Vitronectin expression by Normal ovarian surface epithelial cells: Role in cell adhesion and cell proliferation. Gynecologic Oncology. 1999;**75**(2):254-260

[108] Cannistra SA, Kansas GS, Niloff J, DeFranzo B, Kim Y, Ottensmeier C. Binding of ovarian cancer cells to peritoneal mesothelium in vitro is partly mediated by CD44H. Cancer Research. 1993;**53**(16):3830-3838

[109] Ismail RS, Baldwin RL, Fang J, Browning D, Karlan BY, Gasson JC, et al. Differential gene expression between normal and tumor-derived ovarian epithelial cells. Cancer Research. 2000;**60**(23):6744-6749

[110] Kohn EC, Travers LA, Kassis J, Broome U, Klominek J. Malignant effusions are sources of fibronectin and

other promigratory and proinvasive components. Diagnostic Cytopathology. 2005;**33**(5):300-308

[111] Carduner L, Agniel R, Kellouche S, Picot CR, Blanc-Fournier C, Leroy-Dudal J, et al. Ovarian cancer ascites-derived vitronectin and fibronectin: Combined purification, molecular features and effects on cell response. Biochimica et Biophysica Acta. 2013;**1830**(10):4885-4897

[112] Reuning U. Integrin αvβ3 promotes vitronectin gene expression in human ovarian cancer cells by implicating rel transcription factors. Journal of Cellular Biochemistry. 2011;**112**(7): 1909-1919

[113] Hapke S, Kessler H, Luber B, Benge A, Hutzler P, Höfler H, et al. Ovarian cancer cell proliferation and motility is induced by engagement of integrin alpha(v)beta3/Vitronectin interaction. Biological Chemistry. 2003;**384**(7):1073-1083

[114] Heyman L, Kellouche S, Fernandes J, Dutoit S, Poulain L, Carreiras F. Vitronectin and its receptors partly mediate adhesion of ovarian cancer cells to peritoneal mesothelium in vitro. Tumor Biology. 2008;**29**(4):231-244

[115] Carreiras F, Rigot V, Cruet S, Andre F, Gauduchon P, Marvaldi J. Migration properties of the human ovarian adenocarcinoma cell line IGROV1: Importance of alpha(v)beta3 integrins and vitronectin. International Journal of Cancer. 1999;**80**(2): 285-294

[116] Kenny HA, Kaur S, Coussens LM, Lengyel E. The initial steps of ovarian cancer cell metastasis are mediated by MMP-2 cleavage of vitronectin and fibronectin. The Journal of Clinical Investigation. 2008;**118**(4):1367-1379

[117] Carduner L, Leroy-Dudal J, Picot CR, Gallet O, Carreiras F, Kellouche S. Ascites-induced shift along epithelial-mesenchymal spectrum in ovarian cancer cells: Enhancement of their invasive behavior partly dependant on αv integrins. Clinical & Experimental Metastasis. 2014;**31**(6):675-688

[118] O'Toole S, McGuinness E, Sheppard B, Bonnar J. Plasminogen activators and inhibitors in ovarian adenocarcinomas. International Journal of Gynecological Cancer: Official Journal of the International Gynecological Cancer Society. 1999;**9**(1):61-66

[119] Dolo V, D'Ascenzo S, Violini S, Pompucci L, Festuccia C, Ginestra A, et al. Matrix-degrading proteinases are shed in membrane vesicles by ovarian cancer cells in vivo and in vitro. Clinical & Experimental Metastasis. 1999;**17**(2):131-140

[120] Pedersen N, Schmitt M, Rønne E, Nicoletti MI, Høyer-Hansen G, Conese M, et al. A ligand-free, soluble urokinase receptor is present in the ascitic fluid from patients with ovarian cancer. The Journal of Clinical Investigation. 1993;**92**(5):2160-2167

[121] Tecimer C, Doering DL, Goldsmith LJ, Meyer JS, Abdulhay G, Wittliff JL. Clinical relevance of urokinase-type plasminogen activator, its receptor and inhibitor type 1 in ovarian cancer. International Journal of Gynecological Cancer: Official Journal of the International Gynecological Cancer Society. 2000;**10**(5):372-381

[122] Ahmed N, Riley C, Oliva K, Rice G, Quinn M. Ascites induces modulation of α6β1 integrin and urokinase plasminogen activator receptor expression and associated functions in ovarian carcinoma. British Journal of Cancer. 2005;**92**(8):1475-1485

[123] Clark EA, Brugge JS. Integrins and signal transduction pathways: The road taken. Science (New York, N.Y.). 1995;**268**(5208):233-239

[124] Lengyel E, Wang H, Gum R, Simon C, Wang Y, Boyd D. Elevated urokinase-type plasminogen activator receptor expression in a colon cancer cell line is due to a constitutively activated extracellular signal-regulated kinase-1-dependent signaling cascade. Oncogene. 1997;**14**(21):2563-2573

[125] Sebolt-Leopold JS, Dudley DT, Herrera R, Van Becelaere K, Wiland A, Gowan RC, et al. Blockade of the MAP kinase pathway suppresses growth of colon tumors in vivo. Nature Medicine. 1999;**5**(7):810-816

[126] Agarwal R, Kaye SB. Ovarian cancer: Strategies for overcoming resistance to chemotherapy. Nature Reviews. Cancer. 2003;**3**(7):502-516

[127] Yap TA, Carden CP, Kaye SB. Beyond chemotherapy: Targeted therapies in ovarian cancer. Nature Reviews. Cancer. 2009;**9**(3):167-181

[128] Sawada K, Ohyagi-Hara C, Kimura T, Morishige K. Integrin inhibitors as a therapeutic agent for ovarian cancer. Journal of Oncology. 2012;**2012**:915140

[129] Brooks PC, Clark RA, Cheresh DA. Requirement of vascular integrin alpha v beta 3 for angiogenesis. Science. 1994;**264**(5158):569-571

[130] Montenegro CF, Salla-Pontes CL, Ribeiro JU, Machado AZ, Ramos RF, Figueiredo CC, et al. Blocking alphavbeta3 integrin by a recombinant RGD disintegrin impairs VEGF signaling in endothelial cells. Biochimie. 2012;**94**(8):1812-1820

[131] Kim S, Harris M, Varner JA. Regulation of integrin alpha vbeta 3-mediated endothelial cell migration and angiogenesis by integrin alpha5beta1 and protein kinase a. The Journal of Biological Chemistry. 2000;**275**(43):33920-33928

[132] Jin H, Varner J. Integrins: Roles in cancer development and as treatment targets. British Journal of Cancer. 2004;**90**(3):561-565

[133] Sluiter N, de Cuba E, Kwakman R, Kazemier G, Meijer G, Te Velde EA. Adhesion molecules in peritoneal dissemination: Function, prognostic relevance and therapeutic options. Clinical & Experimental Metastasis. 2016;**33**(5):401-416

[134] Weis SM, Cheresh DA. alphaV integrins in angiogenesis and cancer. Cold Spring Harbor Perspectives in Medicine. 2011;**1**(1):a006478

[135] Brooks PC, Montgomery AM, Rosenfeld M, Reisfeld RA, Hu T, Klier G, et al. Integrin alpha v beta 3 antagonists promote tumor regression by inducing apoptosis of angiogenic blood vessels. Cell. 1994;**79**(7):1157 1164

[136] Voura EB, Ramjeesingh RA, Montgomery AM, Siu CH. Involvement of integrin alpha(v)beta(3) and cell adhesion molecule L1 in transendothelial migration of melanoma cells. Molecular Biology of the Cell. 2001;**12**(9):2699-2710

[137] Cooper CR, Chay CH, Pienta KJ. The role of alpha(v)beta(3) in prostate cancer progression. Neoplasia. 2002;**4**(3):191-194

[138] Rolli M, Fransvea E, Pilch J, Saven A, Felding-Habermann B. Activated integrin alphavbeta3 cooperates with metalloproteinase MMP-9 in regulating migration of metastatic breast cancer cells. Proceedings of the National Academy of

Sciences of the United States of America. 2003;**100**(16):9482-9487

[139] Sloan EK, Pouliot N, Stanley KL, Chia J, Moseley JM, Hards DK, et al. Tumor-specific expression of alphavbeta3 integrin promotes spontaneous metastasis of breast cancer to bone. Breast Cancer Research. 2006;**8**(2):R20

[140] Hapke S, Kessler H, Luber B, Benge A, Hutzler P, Hofler H, et al. Ovarian cancer cell proliferation and motility is induced by engagement of integrin alpha(v)beta3/Vitronectin interaction. Biological Chemistry. 2003;**384**(7):1073-1083

[141] Maubant S, Cruet-Hennequart S, Poulain L, Carreiras F, Sichel F, Luis J, et al. Altered adhesion properties and alphav integrin expression in a cisplatin-resistant human ovarian carcinoma cell line. International Journal of Cancer. 2002;**97**(2):186-194

[142] Landen CN, Kim TJ, Lin YG, Merritt WM, Kamat AA, Han LY, et al. Tumor-selective response to antibody-mediated targeting of alphavbeta3 integrin in ovarian cancer. Neoplasia. 2008;**10**(11):1259-1267

[143] Kim TJ, Landen CN, Lin YG, Mangala LS, Lu C, Nick AM, et al. Combined anti-angiogenic therapy against VEGF and integrin alphaVbeta3 in an orthotopic model of ovarian cancer. Cancer Biology & Therapy. 2009;**8**(23):2263-2272

[144] Kaur S, Kenny HA, Jagadeeswaran S, Zillhardt MR, Montag AG, Kistner E, et al. {beta}3-integrin expression on tumor cells inhibits tumor progression, reduces metastasis, and is associated with a favorable prognosis in patients with ovarian cancer. The American Journal of Pathology. 2009;**175**(5):2184-2196

[145] Reynolds AR, Hart IR, Watson AR, Welti JC, Silva RG, Robinson SD, et al. Stimulation of tumor growth and angiogenesis by low concentrations of RGD-mimetic integrin inhibitors. Nature Medicine. 2009;**15**(4):392-400

[146] Casey RC, Burleson KM, Skubitz KM, Pambuccian SE, Oegema TR Jr, Ruff LE, et al. Beta 1-integrins regulate the formation and adhesion of ovarian carcinoma multicellular spheroids. The American Journal of Pathology. 2001;**159**(6):2071-2080

[147] Ramakrishnan V, Bhaskar V, Law DA, Wong MH, DuBridge RB, Breinberg D, et al. Preclinical evaluation of an anti-alpha5beta1 integrin antibody as a novel anti-angiogenic agent. Journal of Experimental Therapeutics & Oncology. 2006;**5**(4):273-286

[148] Francis SE, Goh KL, Hodivala-Dilke K, Bader BL, Stark M, Davidson D, et al. Central roles of alpha5beta1 integrin and fibronectin in vascular development in mouse embryos and embryoid bodies. Arteriosclerosis, Thrombosis, and Vascular Biology. 2002;**22**(6):927-933

[149] Ricart AD, Tolcher AW, Liu G, Holen K, Schwartz G, Albertini M, et al. Volociximab, a chimeric monoclonal antibody that specifically binds alpha5beta1 integrin: A phase I, pharmacokinetic, and biological correlative study. Clinical Cancer Research. 2008;**14**(23):7924-7929

[150] Burger RA, Brady MF, Bookman MA, Fleming GF, Monk BJ, Huang H, et al. Incorporation of bevacizumab in the primary treatment of ovarian cancer. The New England Journal of Medicine. 2011;**365**(26):2473-2483

[151] Zhou M, Yu P, Qu X, Liu Y, Zhang J. Phase III trials of standard chemotherapy

with or without bevacizumab for ovarian cancer: A meta-analysis. PLoS One. 2013;**8**(12):e81858

[152] Mahmood RD, Morgan RD, Edmondson RJ, Clamp AR, Jayson GC. First-line Management of Advanced High-Grade Serous Ovarian Cancer. Current Oncology Reports. 2020;**22**(6):64

[153] Pilkington-Miksa M, Arosio D, Battistini L, Belvisi L, De Matteo M, Vasile F, et al. Design, synthesis, and biological evaluation of novel cRGD-paclitaxel conjugates for integrin-assisted drug delivery. Bioconjugate Chemistry. 2012;**23**(8):1610-1622

[154] Zhao H, Wang JC, Sun QS, Luo CL, Zhang Q. RGD-based strategies for improving antitumor activity of paclitaxel-loaded liposomes in nude mice xenografted with human ovarian cancer. Journal of Drug Targeting. 2009;**17**(1):10-18

[155] Dougherty TJ, Gomer CJ, Henderson BW, Jori G, Kessel D, Korbelik M, et al. Photodynamic therapy. Journal of the National Cancer Institute. 1998;**90**(12):889-905

[156] Agostinis P, Berg K, Cengel KA, Foster TH, Girotti AW, Gollnick SO, et al. Photodynamic therapy of cancer: An update. CA: A Cancer Journal for Clinicians. 2011;**61**(4):250-281

[157] Celli JP, Spring BQ, Rizvi I, Evans CL, Samkoe KS, Verma S, et al. Imaging and photodynamic therapy: Mechanisms, monitoring, and optimization. Chemical Reviews. 2010;**110**(5):2795-2838

[158] Rizvi I, Nath S, Obaid G, Ruhi MK, Moore K, Bano S, et al. A combination of Visudyne and a lipid-anchored liposomal formulation of benzoporphyrin derivative enhances photodynamic therapy efficacy in a 3D model for ovarian cancer. Photochemistry and Photobiology. 2019;**95**(1):419-429

[159] Bhandari C, Guirguis M, Savan NA, Shrivastava N, Oliveira S, Hasan T, et al. What NIR photodynamic activation offers molecular targeted nanomedicines: Perspectives into the conundrum of tumor specificity and selectivity. Nano Today. 2021;**36**. Article number: 101052

[160] Sorrin AJ, Kemal Ruhi M, Ferlic NA, Karimnia V, Polacheck WJ, Celli JP, et al. Photodynamic therapy and the biophysics of the tumor microenvironment. Photochemistry and Photobiology. 2020;**96**(2):232-259

[161] Liang BJ, Pigula M, Baglo Y, Najafali D, Hasan T, Huang HC. Breaking the selectivity-uptake trade-off of photoimmunoconjugates with nanoliposomal irinotecan for synergistic multi-tier cancer targeting. Journal of Nanobiotechnology. 2020;**18**(1):1

[162] Zhang Y, Zhan X, Xiong J, Peng S, Huang W, Joshi R, et al. Temperature dependent cell death patterns induced by functionalized gold nanoparticle photothermal therapy in melanoma cells. Scientific Reports. 2018;**8**(1):8720

[163] Runnels JM, Chen N, Ortel B, Kato D, Hasan T. BPD-MA-mediated photosensitisation in vitro and in vivo: Cellular adhesion and β1 integrin expression in ovarian cancer cells. British Journal of Cancer. 1999;**80**(7):946-953

[164] Li F, Zhao Y, Mao C, Kong Y, Ming X. RGD-modified albumin Nanoconjugates for targeted delivery of a porphyrin photosensitizer. Molecular Pharmaceutics. 2017;**14**(8):2793-2804

[165] Klein OJ, Yuan H, Nowell NH, Kaittanis C, Josephson L, Evans CL.

An integrin-targeted, highly diffusive construct for photodynamic therapy. Scientific Reports. 2017;**7**(1):13375

[166] Dai J, Li Y, Long Z, Jiang R, Zhuang Z, Wang Z, et al. Efficient near-infrared photosensitizer with aggregation-induced emission for imaging-guided photodynamic therapy in multiple xenograft tumor models. ACS Nano. 2020;**14**(1):854-866

[167] Shaw SK, Schreiber CL, Roland FM, Battles PM, Brennan SP, Padanilam SJ, et al. High expression of integrin alphavbeta3 enables uptake of targeted fluorescent probes into ovarian cancer cells and tumors. Bioorganic & Medicinal Chemistry. 2018;**26**(8):2085-2091

[168] Alvero AB, Kim D, Lima E, Sumi NJ, Lee JS, Cardenas C, et al. Novel approach for the detection of intraperitoneal micrometastasis using an ovarian cancer mouse model. Scientific Reports. 2017;**7**:40989

[169] Harlaar NJ, Kelder W, Sarantopoulos A, Bart J, Themelis G, van Dam GM, et al. Real-time near infrared fluorescence (NIRF) intra-operative imaging in ovarian cancer using an alpha(v)beta(3-)integrin targeted agent. Gynecologic Oncology. 2013;**128**(3):590-595

[170] Aina OH, Marik J, Gandour-Edwards R, Lam KS. Near-infrared optical imaging of ovarian cancer xenografts with novel alpha 3-integrin binding peptide "OA02". Molecular Imaging. 2005;**4**(4):439-447

[171] Zhou H, Xu H, Li X, Lv Y, Ma T, Guo S, et al. Dual targeting hyaluronic acid—RGD mesoporous silica coated gold nanorods for chemo-photothermal cancer therapy. Materials Science & Engineering. C, Materials for Biological Applications. 2017;**81**:261-270

Section 4

Novel Ovarian Cancer Therapeutics

Chapter 5

PARP Inhibitors in the Treatment of Epithelial Ovarian Cancer

Nicola Di Santo, Greta Bagnolini, Yin Wong, Marco Carnelli and Luigi Frigerio

Abstract

Epithelial ovarian cancer (EOC), the most lethal gynecologic malignancy in the western world, has been historically treated with surgery followed by chemotherapy. Poly (ADP-ribose) polymerase (PARP) inhibitors are one of the most active new targeted therapies for the treatment of EOC. PARPis' mechanism of action relies on their ability to interfere with DNA repair events leading ultimately to cell death, the biological concept known as synthetic lethality. Initially developed as maintenance therapy in patients with a response after platinum-based chemotherapy in a recurrent setting, PARPis are now approved as the frontline treatment strategy. The aim of this chapter is to examine PARPis' antineoplastic activity and the clinical development studies that lead to their approval, as well as the safety and the management of adverse events associated with this new class of drugs. Lastly, the rational considerations for the use of PARPis in the frontline setting are discussed.

Keywords: ovarian cancer, poly (ADP-ribose) polymerase inhibitors (PARP inhibitors), maintenance therapy, homologous recombination pathway, *BRCA* mutation, hematologic toxicities

1. Introduction

Epithelial ovarian cancer (EOC) is the second most common and the most lethal gynecologic malignancy responsible worldwide for ≈ 207,000 deaths [1]. EOC affects mainly postmenopausal women and is typically diagnosed at an advanced stage due to the absence of specific symptoms compounded with no effective early screening modalities that allow to detect the disease when it is localized [2, 3].

Several studies have demonstrated that advanced EOC represents a heterogeneous group of malignancies with complex molecular and genetic features associated with specific pathogenic pathways alteration and phenotypic clinical behavior [4]. High-grade serous ovarian carcinomas (HGSOC) represent the most common histotype and are linked to poor prognosis [4]. The vast majority of HGSOC arises from the fallopian tube (FT) as a precursor known as serous tubal intraepithelial carcinoma [5]. Moreover, several findings suggested that FT and primary peritoneal cancer (PPC) share the same pathobiology and genetic aberrations associated with HGSOC. As such, patients diagnosed with "pelvis serous carcinoma" should be considered as collectively having the same disease and, therefore, they should receive uniform treatment options [5].

Furthermore, the Cancer Genome Atlas (TCGA) project has identified that approximately 50% of HGSOC exhibits defects in homologous recombination repair (HRR) pathway, which is major biochemical machinery for the repair of DNA double-strand breaks (DSBs) in mammalian cells [6]. DSBs represent the most serious manifestation of DNA damage because, if left unrepaired, they can lead to genomic instability, which is considered one of the main features of carcinogenesis [7]. Given that breast cancer gene (BRCA)1 and (BRCA)2 are the tumor suppressor genes (wild-type BRCA allele is lost during tumorigenesis) involved at different stages of HRR, carriers of deleterious heterozygous germline mutations in the BRCA1 and BRCA2 genes have significantly elevated risks of developing breast, ovarian, and other cancers [7]. At the same time, tumors that exhibit homologous recombination deficiency (HRD) are susceptible to specific systemic treatments, including poly ADP-ribose polymerase (PARP) inhibitors (PARPis) [8].

Poly(ADP-ribose)polymerases (PARPs) are a family of nuclear ubiquitous enzymes, which regulate the biological functions of a variety of proteins by catalyzing their posttranslational modification, named PARylation, using NAD+ as substrate [9]. By post-transcriptionally modifying multiple proteins, PARPs act as signal transducers, contributing to the regulation of various cellular functions including the signaling pathway that leads to the resolution of DNA strand breaks. In this context, PARPs play as promoters of genomic integrity and stability, activating different mechanisms for DNA repair, stabilizing replication forks, and modeling the chromatin structure [10].

PARP1 is the most abundant and studied member of the PARP family, accounting for 80–90% of total PARP activity in the cell, and it is also known as the major PAR-producing enzyme in eukaryotes [11–13]. PARP1 is centrally involved in the early response to cellular oxidative and genotoxic stress, to which cells are constantly exposed [10]. In this context, PARP1 acts as a crucial DNA damage sensor, participating in the DNA damage response (DDR), the network of molecular pathways that maintain the genomic integrity by recognizing DNA damages and orchestrating their repair [14]. In DDR, PARP1's first action is to trigger the repair of DNA single-strand breaks (SSBs) to ensure cellular genomic stability. Indeed, if not repaired, SSBs are likely to be converted, during DNA replication, into DSBs, the most harmful form of DNA damage that led to the genomic instability, eventually responsible for the development of many diseases, including cancer [10, 15].

In addition, PARP1 promotes the repair of DNA DSBs through the high-fidelity homologous recombination (HR), by activating and recruiting multiple proteins such as ATM, Mre11, and Nbs11 to DSB lesions, and simultaneously inactivating DNA-dependent protein kinases that favor the more error-prone nonhomologous end-joining (NHEJ) [16].

Suppression of PARP1 leads to the accumulation of unrepaired DNA SSBs and the stalling of replication forks [17]. The persistence of SSBs culminates in the collapse of stalled replication forks into highly cytotoxic DSBs. HR is considered the highest fidelity machinery to repair DSBs and indispensable to maintain the genomic integrity. HR, as a complex mechanism, involves a large number of proteins that operate from the DSBs detection to the effective DNA repair. In this context, BRCA1 and BRCA2 are crucial players to guarantee HR high efficiency. Indeed, both proteins interact with many HR effectors, participating in the DSB detection and guiding the formation of the complex that effectively repairs the DNA strand. BRCA2 is even more important since it is responsible for the recruitment and loading onto the DNA strand of RAD51, the recombinase, defined as the catalytic core of HR, that guides homology search and strand invasion.

In case of PARP inhibition, HR acts as a compensatory pathway to maintain the genomic integrity and guarantee cell survival [16]. Normal cells are BRCA-proficient, thus able to efficiently repair DSBs and survive under PARP inhibition. On the contrary, cancers harboring BRCA1 or BRCA2 mutations become HR-defective and highly vulnerable to the effects of PARP inhibition, facing a genomic instability that turns into cell death [18]. This relationship has been defined as synthetic lethality (SL) and it has been exploited as a strategy to selectively target cancers with somatic and germline BRCA1 and BRCA2 mutations [18]. The concept of SL was originally derived from genetic studies on gene-to-gene interactions and their consequent impact on cell viability. According to this genetic principle, two genes are synthetic lethal if their simultaneous mutation causes cell death, while the mutation of either gene alone is compatible with cell viability. (**Figure 1**).

This SL relationship can be explained by the presence of a buffering effect, which links two genes and is lost in case of simultaneous mutation. The SL concept can be extended to proteins encoded by synthetic lethal genes and, in turn, to the cellular pathways. According to this, SL has been exploited for drug discovery to selectively treat cancers, harboring a specific gene mutation, with drugs targeting the synthetic lethal partner. Notably, taking advantage of a mutation present only in cancer cells, SL approach promises to be selective, killing cancer cells while sparing normal ones.

The evidence of a synthetic lethal interaction between PARP inhibition and BRCA1/2 mutation suggested a clinical strategy to treat cancers with loss-of-function mutations in either BRCA1 or BRCA2 genes with PARPis as drugs [14, 16]. PARP1 is the primary target of clinically used PARPis. Initially, PARP1 inhibitors were developed to be used as potentiators of DNA damaging chemo- or radiotherapeutic agents [14, 19]. Later, PARPis revealed their potential as single agents in the treatment of BRCAness tumors with an HR-defective condition. BRCAness refers to tumors with specific genomic signatures (other than BRCA mutation) that cause HR-deficiency and thus susceptibility to SL of PARPis [20]. PARPis block the catalytic activity of PARP1 by directly binding to the NAD+ pocket, responsible for the synthesis of PAR chains. For this reason, the originally proposed mechanism of action (MOA) to explain the SL effect, described PARPis as direct inhibitors of the PARylation, which causes the impairment of DNA repair proteins and the phenocopying effect of deleting PARP1 [19]. Indeed, persistent unrepaired DNA breaks can cause the collapse of replication forks with the formation of DSBs, not repaired by HR-deficient cells. However, the most credited MOA of PARPis is their ability to trap PARP1 on DNA strand, ultimately preventing its release from the DNA strand by the inhibition of autoPARylation and PARP1 conformational change. The trapped PARP1 acts as an obstacle, causing unstable replication forks and consequent accumulation of DNA lesions, which are eventually repaired by error-prone mechanisms in HR-deficient

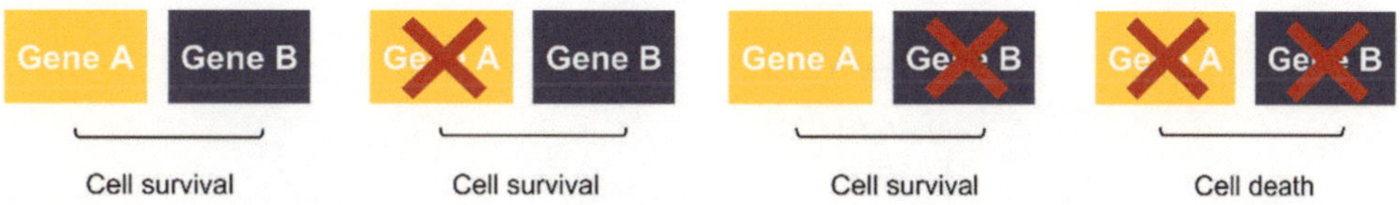

Figure 1.
Concept of synthetic lethality.

cells [19]. This mechanism explains the PARPis cytotoxic effect and most likely accounts for the SL effect in BRCAness tumors.

This chapter examines the clinical development studies, which lead to PARPis approval, the safety and the management of adverse events associated to this new class of drugs, and rational consideration that should guide the use of PARPis in the frontline setting.

2. PARPis and clinical trials

Currently, three PARPis are approved for the treatment of EOC: olaparib, rucaparib, and niraparib. All these drugs are available for the management of recurrent disease as monotherapies, whereas only olaparib and niraparib are approved as frontline maintenance options after a response to platinum-based chemotherapy. Lastly, olaparib is the only approved drug in combination with bevacizumab as a first-line maintenance strategy for a subset of patients whose cancer is associated with HRD status (**Table 1**).

2.1 Recurrent setting

2.1.1 Maintenance therapy in the recurrent setting

Lynparza® (olaparib) is a first-in-class, small molecule, PARPi approved initially as monotherapy for maintenance treatment of patients in response to their most recent platinum-based regimen in olaparib (capsule formulation) in platinum-sensitive, relapsed, BRCA-mutated HGSOC in the EU based on the results of Study 19. [21] In 2014, there were no agents for maintenance treatment of EOC after a response to platinum-containing regimens, and standard of care (SOC) was not clearly established in this setting.

Agent	Maintenance	Later line treatment
Olaparib	Study 19 (EU) • Recurrent	Study 42, SOLO-3 (US) • BRCAm
	SOLO-2 (US) • Recurrent	
	SOLO-1 (US, EU) • BRCAm front-line	
	PAOLA-1 (US, EU) • HRD front-line	
Rucaparib	ARIEL3 (US, EU) • Recurrent	Study 10, ARIEL2, ARIEL4 (EU) • BRCAm
Niraparib	NOVA (US, EU) • Recurrent	QUADRA (US) • HRD
	PRIMA (US, EU) • Frontline	

Table 1.
Current PARPi approved indications in ovarian cancer.

Preliminary studies indicated the olaparib exerted anti-cancer activity in BRCA-negative tumor having a defect in the HR pathway other than related to BRCA mutation (BRACAness phenotype) [22]. Upon these premises, the aim of phase II Study 19 was designed to assess efficacy and safety of olaparib monotherapy as maintenance treatment in patients with platinum-sensitive, relapsed, HGSOC who had a response to their most recent platinum-based chemotherapy [23]. No prospective BRCA testing was required for eligibility for this study, which enrolled 265 patients who had received two or more platinum-based regimens and had a partial or complete response to their most recent platinum-based regimen. Patients were randomly assigned to receive olaparib (400 mg twice daily) or placebo until the primary endpoint progression-free survival (PFS) defined as the time from randomization (on completion of chemotherapy) until the objective assessment of disease progression according to response evaluation criteria in solid tumors (RECIST) guidelines or death. In terms of efficacy results, median PFS in study 19 was significantly longer with olaparib than with placebo (8.4 months vs. 4.8 months; hazard ratio [HR] for progression or death, 0.35; 95%: confidence interval [CI], 0.25 to 0.49; $P < 0.001$) [23].

Furthermore, a prespecified exploratory analysis of all efficacy endpoints performed according to BRCA mutation status demonstrated that patients with a BRCA mutation had the greatest PFS benefit from treatment with olaparib maintenance therapy compared with placebo. For patients with a BRCA mutation, median PFS was significantly longer in the olaparib group than in the placebo group (11.2 months [95% CI 8.3–not calculable] vs. 4.3 months [3.0–5.4]; HR 0.18 [95% CI 0.10–0.31]; $p < 0.0001$) [24]. In December 2014, olaparib was approved in the EU for the maintenance treatment of adults with platinum-sensitive, relapsed, HGSOC, FT, and PPC who are in complete or partial response to platinum-based chemotherapy and BRCA mutation-positive (germline and/or somatic).

To confirm olaparib benefits in the same setting using tablets as opposed to the previous capsule formulation, the double-blinded, randomized, and placebo-controlled phase III SOLO-2 trial was planned. This study enrolled 295 platinum-sensitive relapsed patients with high-grade serous or endometrioid EOC, PT, or PPC, preselected for BRCA1/BRCA2 mutations who were in response to their most recent platinum-based chemotherapy after ≥2 lines of treatment. Participants were randomized 2:1 to maintenance olaparib (300 mg twice daily; tablet) or placebo. The primary endpoint for this study was investigator-assessed PFS. The trial met its primary endpoint with a median PFS of 19.1 months vs. 5.5 months (HR 0.30; 95% CI 0.22 to 0.41; $P < 0.0001$), substantially exceeding the efficacy results seen in Study 19 [25]. Despite SOLO-2 study enrolled only patients with BRCA mutations, based upon the combined results of both Study 19 and SOLO-2 US Food and Drug Administration (FDA) in 2017 and European Medicines Agency (EMA) in 2018 granted approval to olaparib for the maintenance treatment regardless of BRCA mutation status [26].

Zejula® (niraparib) is an oral, small molecule inhibitor of PARP enzymes, including PARP-1 and PARP-2 [27]. After niraparib 300 mg demonstrated preliminary antitumor activity in ovarian cancer patients in phase 1 dose-escalation study, phase III NOVA trial sought to establish the efficacy and safety of niraparib in patients with platinum-sensitive, recurrent, histologically confirmed ovarian cancer as maintenance treatment following complete or partial response to platinum-based chemotherapy [28]. Different from SOLO-2 trial, NOVA study enrolled two independent cohorts based on the presence or absence of a germline BRCA (gBRCA) mutation (gBRCAm) according to BRCA analysis testing (Myriad Genetics, Inc.) from tumor and blood samples. In each cohort (n = 203 for gBRCAm cohort and n = 350 non-gBRCAm cohort), patients were randomly assigned to receive 300 mg of niraparib once daily or placebo in 28-day cycles until disease progression or unacceptable toxicity. Primary endpoint was PFS in intent-to-treat (ITT) analyses of the three predefined primary efficacy populations namely gBRCAm cohort, the HRD-positive subgroup of the non-gBRCAmcohort, and the overall non-gBRCAm cohort. Patients in the niraparib group had a significantly longer median PFS than did those in the placebo group; 21.0 vs. 5.5 months in the gBRCAm cohort (HR, 0.27; 95% CI, 0.17–0.41) and 12.9 months vs. 3.8 months in the non-gBRCAm cohort for patients who had tumors with HRD (HR, 0.38; 95% CI, 0.24–0.59). Finally, the median PFS also favored the niraparib group in the overall non-gBRCAm cohort, 9.3 months vs. 3.9 months (HR ratio, 0.45; 95% CI, 0.34–0.61; $P < 0.001$ for all three comparisons) [28].

The overall results of this study indicated that, among patients with platinum-sensitive, recurrent ovarian cancer, the median duration of PFS was significantly longer among those receiving niraparib compared to those receiving placebo. In March 2017, niraparib received its first FDA and EMA approval for the maintenance treatment of adult patients with recurrent EOC, FT, or PPC who are in a complete or partial response to platinum-based chemotherapy regardless of BRCA mutations or HRD status [27].

Rubraca® (rucaparib) is an oral, small molecule inhibitor of PARP enzymes, including PARP-1, −2, and − 3 [29]. Like the other two PARPis, rucaparib was demonstrated to exert synthetic lethality in cells with HRD [29]. Data of efficacy as maintenance treatment of recurrent EOC was established in phase III ARIEL-3 study, where 564 patients with recurrent platinum-sensitive, high-grade serous or endometrioid ovarian carcinoma had completed at least two platinum-based chemotherapy regimens with response to the last regimen were included [30]. Patients were randomly assigned to receive rucaparib 600 mg twice daily or a placebo after stratification by HRD status, latest progression-free interval, and response to the latest platinum-based regimen. HRD combined tumor BRCA status as well as the percentage of genome-wide loss of heterozygosity (LOH) with the use of Foundation Medicine's T5 next-generation sequencing (NGS) assay.

For patients with BRCA mutations, median PFS in the rucaparib group was 16.6 months compared to 5.4 months in the placebo group (HR 0.23; 95% CI 0.16–0.34; $p < 0.0001$). In patients with HRD tumors, patients receiving rucaparib also had improved PFS compared to placebo (13.6 months vs. 5.4 months; HR 0.32; 95% CI 0.24–0.42; $p < 0.0001$). In the ITT population, the median PFS was 10.8 months in the rucaparib group vs. 5.4 months in the placebo group (HR 0.36; 95% CI 0.30–0.45; $p < 0.0001$) [30]. Based on these data, in 2018, the FDA and EMA granted rucaparib a new indication concerning maintenance treatment for platinum-sensitive relapsed high-grade epithelial ovarian cancer in patients who are in response to platinum-based chemotherapy regardless of BRCA or HRD status [30].

2.1.2 Treatment of recurrent epithelial ovarian cancer

In the US, the first indication for the clinical use of PARP inhibitors in EOC was given for the treatment setting (non-maintenance) of recurrent disease. In 2014, under FDA's accelerated approval pathway, olaparib received its first indication for the treatment of women with recurrent ovarian cancer with gBRCAm who received three or more prior lines of chemotherapy [31]. This approval was based on the analysis of 137 patients from Study 42 which included subjects with measurable

BRCA-deficient recurrent disease treated with a median of 3.4 prior lines of chemotherapy [32]. The objective response rate (ORR) for patients in this cohort with measurable disease was 34% (95% CI, 26–42%) and the median duration of response was 7.9 months (95% CI, 5.6–9.6 months). Of note, this accelerated approval was not restricted to either the platinum-sensitive or platinum-resistant disease setting. The justification is the assumption that olaparib would have a better response rate and favorable safety profile as compared with available single-agent chemotherapeutic options given usually in this setting [31]. Along with the drug, the FDA also approved a molecular companion diagnostic test, BRACAnalysis CDx (Myriad Genetics, Inc.) to detect the presence of gBRCA mutations in blood samples [31].

Accelerated approvals were contingent on the results of phase III confirmatory trial SOLO-3. This open-label study was conducted to compare olaparib with non-platinum chemotherapy in patients with gBRCAm platinum-sensitive relapsed ovarian cancer who had received at least 2 prior lines of platinum-based chemotherapy [33]. Approximately 266 patients were randomly assigned 2:1 to olaparib 300 mg twice a day or physician's choice (PC) single-agent nonplatinum chemotherapy (pegylated liposomal doxorubicin, paclitaxel, gemcitabine, or topotecan). The primary end point was ORR in the measurable disease analysis set assessed by blinded independent central review (BICR). The key secondary end point was PFS assessed by BICR in the ITT population. The BICR-assessed ORR was 72.2% with olaparib versus 51.4% with PC, for an odds ratio of 2.53 (95% CI 1.40–4.58; P = 0.002). Median PFS was 13.4 months with olaparib versus 9.2 months with chemotherapy (HR 0.62, 95% CI 0.43–0.91; P = 0.013) [33]. As of August 2022, the manufacturer of olaparib, AstraZeneca (AZ) has released a Dear HCP Letter informing HCPs that a recent subgroup analysis indicated a potential detrimental effect on OS for olaparib compared to the chemotherapy control arm in SOLO3. AZ is having active discussions with FDA about revisions to the olaparib US prescribing information label and are planning to voluntarily withdraw the late line treatment indication. At the time of publishing, olaparib still holds an active indication for late line treatment [34].

Additionally, rucaparib received FDA accelerated approval in 2016 for treatment of recurrent BRCA-associated EOC based on combined data from two single-arm trials Study 10 and ARIEL2 [35]. The combined analyses included 106 patients with BRCA mutations (germline or somatic) and advanced EOC who had received at least two prior platinum-based chemotherapy regimens. The ORR for treatment with rucaparib 600 mg orally twice a day was 54%, with a median duration of response (DOR) of 9.2 months. As expected, ORR was greatest for those with platinum-sensitive disease (66%; 95% CI: 54–76%) and lowest in platinum-refractory patients (0%; 95% CI: 0–41%). Rucaparib received accelerated approval based on ORR and DOR seen in phase II trials. At the same time, approval of a companion diagnostic test, FoundationFocus CDx $_{BRCA}$ (Foundation Medicine, Inc.) to detect tumor BRCA1 and BRCA2 mutations (germline and/or somatic) was granted [36].

Continued approval of rucaparib in this indication was contingent upon of demonstration of clinical benefit in confirmatory phase 3 trial, ARIEL4 conducted in germline or somatic BRCA mutated patients with relapsed, HGSOC, FT, or PPC that had received at least 2 prior chemotherapy regimens, with at least 1 of which being platinum-based. Treatment with rucaparib was administered at 600 mg twice daily in the investigational arm (n = 233), and in the control arm (n = 116), weekly paclitaxel was given for those who were platinum-resistant or partially sensitive, and platinum-based chemotherapy monotherapy or doublet regimen was given to those who were fully sensitive to platinum. The investigator-assessed median PFS in the efficacy population was 7.4 months (95% CI,

7.3–9.1) with rucaparib in comparison with 5.7 months (95% CI, 5.5–7.3) with chemotherapy (HR, 0.64; 95% CI, 0.49–0.84; P = 0.001). In the ITT population, the median PFS was the same at 7.4 months (95% CI, 6.7–7.9) and 5.7 months (95% CI, 5.5–6.7) in the rucaparib and chemotherapy arms, respectively, but showed a hazard ratio of 0.67 (95% CI, 0.52–0.86; P = 0.0017) [37]. As of June 2022, the manufacturer of rucaparib, Clovis has released a Dear HCP Letter informing HCPs that they have voluntarily withdrawn rucaparib's late line treatment indication in consultation with FDA after a detrimental effect of OS was observed for rucaparib compared to the chemotherapy control arm in the ARIEL-4 trial. Clovis has confirmed they have voluntarily requested the withdrawal of the same BRCAm OC treatment indication in EU. At the time of publishing, Rubraca's indication in later line treatment is still active in EU [38].

Lastly, the role of niraparib in later lines of treatment of patients with relapsed EOC was assessed in a single-arm study [39]. QUADRA was a multicenter, open-label, single-arm study that evaluated the safety and efficacy of niraparib in 463 patients with metastatic, relapsed, HGSOC, FT, or PPC, who were treated previously with at least 3 lines of chemotherapy. QUADRA met its primary endpoint: ORR was 24% (95% CI 16–34%) with the median DOR being 8.3 months. Of note, niraparib demonstrated efficacy beyond patients with BRCA mutation; within the cohort of 35 patients

Trial name	Patients (n) and randomization	Median PFS duration (primary endpoint and biomarker subgroups)
SOLO-1 [40]	391 (olaparib vs. placebo maintenance)	All patients have *BRCA1/2* mutations • Not reached vs. 13.8 months; HR 0.30, 95% CI 0.23–0.41; p < 0.001
PAOLA-1 [41]	806 (olaparib plus bevacizumab vs. placebo plus bevacizumab)	• ITT: 22.1 months vs. 16.6 months (HR 0.59, 95% CI 0.49–0.72; p < 0.001) • HRD-positive: 37.2 months vs. 17.7 months (HR 0.33, 95% CI 0.25–0.45) • HRD-negative: 16.6 months vs. 16.2 months (HR 1.00, 95% CI 0.75–1.35)
PRIMA [42]	733 (niraparib vs. placebo maintenance)	• HRD-positive: 21.9 months vs. 10.4 months (HR 0.43, 95% CI 0.31–0.59; p < 0.001) • ITT: 13.8 months vs. 8.2 months (HR 0.62, 95% CI 0.50–0.76; p < 0.001) • HRD-negative: 8.1 months vs. 5.4 months (HR 0.68, 95% CI 0.49–0.94)
VELIA [43]	1140 (chemotherapy only [control] vs. veliparib combination only vs. veliparib throughout)	Veliparib throughout vs. control: • BRCA1/2-mutated: 34.7 months and 22.0 months (HR 0.44, 95% CI 0.28–0.68; p < 0.001) • HRD-positive: 31.9 months and 20.5 months (HR 0.57, 95% CI 0.43–0.76; p < 0.001) • ITT: 23.5 months and 17.3 months (HR 0.68, 95% CI 0.56–0.83; p < 0.001) • HRD-negative: HR 0.81, 95% CI 0.60–1.09
ATHENA-MONO [44]	538 (rucaparib vs. placebo maintenance)	• HRD-positive: 28.7 months vs. 11.3 months (HR 0.47; 95% CI: 0.31–0.72; p = 0.0004) • ITT:20.2 months vs. 9.2 months (HR, 0.52; 95% CI, 0.40–0.68; P < .0001) • HRD-negative: 12.1 months vs. 9.1 months (HR, 0.65; 95% CI, 0.45–0.95)

Table 2.
Results of Phase III Trials for PARPi maintenance in front-line setting.

with non-BRCA-mutated tumors who were HRD-positive and platinum-sensitive, the ORR was 20%. As a result, in October 2019, niraparib received FDA approval as a monotherapy treatment for recurrent EOC who had received three or more prior chemotherapy regimens in the context of HRD-positive tumors. HRD positive status is defined by either a deleterious, suspected deleterious BRCA mutation, or genomic instability, and who has progressed more than six months after responding to the last platinum-based chemotherapy [27].

2.2 Frontline maintenance treatment

After the positive results achieved for relapsed disease, four Phase III studies investigated the role of PARP inhibitors as maintenance therapy following platinum-based chemotherapy in newly diagnosed advanced EOC (**Table 2**). The outcomes of these studies redesigned the treatment landscape of EOC offering several therapeutic options to patients in the frontline setting.

The evidence for the use of olaparib maintenance as a SOC for women with newly diagnosed advanced ovarian cancer and BRCA mutation is derived from the result of SOLO-1 trial [40]. In this double-blind, placebo-controlled, multicenter trial newly diagnosed stage III or IV, high-grade serous or endometrioid ovarian, FT, PPC, and germline BRCA mutations in complete response (CR) or partial response (PR) after platinum-based chemotherapy were randomized 2:1 to olaparib at 300 mg twice daily (n = 260) versus placebo (n = 131) for up to 2 years or until disease progression. At the primary analysis cutoff date of May 2018 the median PFS for patients treated with olaparib was not reached compared to 13.8 months for patients treated with placebo (HR, 0.30; 95% CI, 0.23–0.41; P < 0.001). Based on this data, in December 2018, olaparib received regulatory approval in the 1st-line maintenance setting for BRCAm advanced ovarian cancer in the US. The same indication has been granted in the EU in June 2019 [45].

Longer-term follow-up data from SOLO-1 revealed that the benefit of olaparib was sustained after treatment was stopped, with 48% of women treated with olaparib remaining progression-free for 5 years compared to 21% of placebo patients. Median PFS was 56·0 months (95% CI 41·9-not reached) for olaparib versus 13·8 months (11·1–18·2) for placebo (HR 0.33 [95% CI 0.25–0.43]) [46].

Shortly after, niraparib also demonstrated to improve PFS as first-line maintenance therapy vs. placebo in patients with newly diagnosed advanced ovarian cancer at high risk for relapse who responded to platinum-based chemotherapy irrespective of HRD status. The PRIMA trial was a randomized, double-blind, phase 3 trial in which participants after achieving a response to platinum-based chemotherapy were assigned in a 2:1 ratio to receive niraparib or placebo once daily [42]. At the onset of the trial, niraparib was administered at a fixed dose of 300 mg once daily. To improve safety and tolerability, following a protocol amendment, the dosage of niraparib was reduced to 200 mg once daily in patients with a body weight of <77 kg and/or a platelet count of <150,000/mcL at baseline. The primary end point was PFS in patients who had tumors with HRD and in the overall population, as determined by hierarchical testing. HRD was defined as the presence of a deleterious BRCA gene mutation and/or a myChoice test (Myriad Genetics, Inc.) score of ≥42 out of 100 (higher scores indicate higher levels of genomic abnormality). HR-proficient namely HRD-negative patients or patients who had an undetermined HRD status were included in the overall population. In the overall population, niraparib demonstrated a median PFS of 13.8 months compared with 8.2 months in patients who received placebo, leading to a 38% reduction in the risk of disease, progression, or death

(HR, 0.62; 95% CI, 0.50–0.76; P < 0.001). In a subgroup of patients whose tumors were positive for HRD, the median PFS with niraparib was 21.9 months compared with 10.4 months for placebo (HR, 0.43; 95% CI, 0.31–0.59; P < 0.001). In addition, in HRD-negative the median PFS with niraparib was 8.1 months compared with 5.4 months for placebo (HR 0.68, 95% CI 0.49–0.94) [42].

In April 2020, niraparib was approved by the FDA for frontline maintenance in patients with advanced epithelial ovarian, fallopian tube, or primary peritoneal cancer who experience complete or partial response to platinum-based chemotherapy [47]. A few months later also EMA granted the approval of niraparib for the same indication [48].

Two randomized phase 3 trials combining bevacizumab with a carboplatin–paclitaxel doublet for newly diagnosed EOC have demonstrated to improve PFS [49, 50]. Bevacizumab received regulatory approval for stage IIIB, IIIC, and IV as induction, in combination with chemotherapy, followed by maintenance monotherapy ovarian cancer in 2011 in the EU. On the contrary, FDA approved bevacizumab only in 2018 in this setting. Under the hypothesis that bevacizumab could cause hypoxia-induced HRD in the tumor and thereby increase sensitivity to PARPis, PAOLA-1 trial was designed to compare maintenance olaparib in combination with bevacizumab versus placebo plus bevacizumab [41]. Notably, PAOLA-1 was the only trial to include an active maintenance comparator in the first-line maintenance setting. The study enrolled 806 newly diagnosed advanced EOC patients who had no evidence of residual disease and were in clinical complete or partial response after receiving chemotherapy plus bevacizumab, regardless of surgical status and BRCAm status. Participants were randomized, to either bevacizumab (continued for 15 months) alone or olaparib (continued for up to 24 months) and bevacizumab.

In the overall population, a statistically significant improvement in median PFS (primary endpoint) for olaparib plus bevacizumab vs. bevacizumab alone (22.1 vs. 16.6 months, HR = 0.59; 95% CI = 0.49–0.72; P < 0.001) was observed. In the predefined subgroups, substantial PFS benefit was observed with the combination treatment vs. bevacizumab in the HRD population (including BRCA1/2 mutant; 37.2 vs. 17.7 months; HR = 0.33; 95% CI = 0.25–0.45). Further, for the patients that were HRD positive but did not have a BRCA mutation, the median PFS was 28.1 months in the combination arm versus 16.6 months in the bevacizumab arm (HR 0.43, 95% CI 0.28–0.66). Interestingly, the median PFS for the patients who tested negative for HRD was similar between the olaparib group and placebo; 16.6 months vs. 16.2 months (HR 1.00, 95% CI 0.75–1.35) [41].

Given that a superior clinical benefit was not demonstrated with olaparib versus placebo in HR proficient patients, FDA and EMA approved olaparib in combination with bevacizumab for the maintenance treatment of adult patients with advanced EOC, FT, or PPC who are in CR or PR to front line platinum-based chemotherapy and whose cancer is associated with HRD status defined by either a deleterious or suspected deleterious BRCA mutation and/or genomic instability [21, 49].

During PARPis development, the attempts of combining these agents with cytotoxic chemotherapy have presented several challenges due to the overlapping toxicities such as myelosuppression, which made it difficult to establish appropriate dosages [52].

Among the similar same class of compounds, veliparib is considered to be less potent PARP catalytic inhibitor and a less potent DNA-PARP trapper [51]. Given this intrinsic pharmacological feature, veliparib is the only PARPi studied in combination with platinum-based chemotherapy in EOC in the first line setting. The aim of phase

III VELIA trial is to assess the safety and efficacy of veliparib in both the frontline induction (with carboplatin/paclitaxel chemotherapy) and maintenance phases in HGSOC, FT, or PPC [43].

A total of 1140 patients were enrolled and randomized into 3 arms. The first arm received carboplatin and paclitaxel plus placebo followed by placebo maintenance. Arm 2 received carboplatin and paclitaxel plus veliparib followed by placebo maintenance. The third arm was the most significant for improving PFS meeting the endpoint of the trial. Patients in this arm received carboplatin and paclitaxel plus veliparib followed by veliparib maintenance. Of note, after the 6 cycles of combination chemotherapy, patients received an additional 30 cycles of maintenance therapy with either placebo or veliparib 300 mg twice daily escalating to 400 mg twice daily if tolerated. In contrast with PRIMA, PAOLA-1, and SOLO1, the PFS (primary endpoint) of the VELIA study was calculated from the start of chemotherapy. In addition, due to the study design, patients with stable disease (not only subjects with CR or PR after carboplatin and paclitaxel) received single-agent veliparib maintenance [43].

In the primary analyses of the VELIA trial, the addition of veliparib to carboplatin-paclitaxel and continuation as maintenance therapy resulted in statistically significant improvements in PFS in the BRCAm, HRD, and ITT populations. Using myChoice assay (Myriad Genetics, Inc.), a score of ≥33 was considered to indicate HRD status. To increase the sensitivity of detecting a response to PARPi, threshold score was revised from 42 to 33. The overall study results showed a significant PFS benefit for the veliparib throughout arm versus the control arm. The median PFS for the induction and maintenance phases combined in the ITT population was 23.5 months compared with 17.3 months in the control arm (HR, 0.68; 95% CI, 0.56–0.83; $P < 0.001$). As expected, the magnitude of the clinical benefit was larger in subjects with BRCA mutations with a median PFS of 34.7 months compared with 22.0 months for veliparib and placebo, respectively (HR, 0.44; 95% CI, 0.28–0.68; $P < 0.001$). Lastly, the median PFS in the subgroup of patients with HRD was 31.9 months for the veliparib throughout arm versus 20.5 months for the chemotherapy-alone arm, with an HR of 0.57 (95% CI, 0.43–0.76; $P < 0.001$). Given that no benefit in terms of PFS was obtained in any stratified biomarker population looking at combination chemotherapy only arm vs. control arm these results suggest that the benefit from veliparib is gained with maintenance therapy extension [43]. Currently, no health regulatory agency has approved veliparib in any setting of advance EOC.

Finally, very recently, rucaparib monotherapy demonstrated a significant improvement in PFS when given as first-line maintenance in EOC following treatment of platinum-based chemotherapy. In the phase III ATHENA-MONO trial, 538 patients with high-grade ovarian, FT, or PPC were allocated in 4:1 fashion to either rucaparib or placebo. Rucaparib/placebo continued for a maximum of 24 months or until disease progression, unacceptable toxicity, or death [44]. The primary endpoint was investigator-assessed PFS, which was analyzed in the HRD-positive subgroup including BRCAm or BRCA wild type/LOH-high and the ITT population.

In the ITT population, the median PFS was 20.2 months with rucaparib compared to 9.2 months with placebo (HR, 0.52; 95% CI, 0.40–0.68; $P < 0.0001$). Further, the median PFS for the HRD-positive patient population treated with rucaparib was 28.7 months vs. 11.3 months among those who received placebo ($p = 0.0004$) with HR 0.47 (95% CI: 0.31–0.72). Finally, in the HRD-negative subgroup, the median PFS was 12.1 months in the rucaparib group and 9.1 months in the placebo group (HR, 0.65; 95% CI, 0.45–0.95) underscoring the benefit that rucaparib can provide to women with EOC irrespective of HRD status [44]. To date, rucaparib has not received approval in the first-line ovarian cancer maintenance setting.

3. Safety and management of adverse events of PARPis

3.1 Dosing, administration, and drug interactions

PARP inhibitors are available in oral dosing forms (tablet or capsule). The starting dose of olaparib is at 300 mg twice daily and rucaparib at 600 mg twice daily [51, 54]. Niraparib is the only once-daily PARPi with an individualized starting dose based on weight (< or ≥ 77 kg) and/or platelet count (< or ≥ 150,000/mcl) at 200 mg or 300 mg for first-line maintenance advanced EOC indication [47, 48] and 300 mg once daily for all other indications [47]. Of note, approximately 15% of patients in the NOVA study weighed <58 kg and the incidence of grade 3 or 4 adverse events was higher in the patients with lower body weight (<58 kg). As such, a starting dose of niraparib 200 mg for patients weighing less than 58 kg may be considered [48].

Olaparib may be dose adjusted to 200 mg twice daily in patients with moderate renal impairment [21, 51] and the use of olaparib is not recommended in patients with severe renal impairment [21] whereas niraparib may be dose adjusted to a starting dose of 200 mg once daily for moderate hepatic impairment [47]. No starting dose adjustment is recommended for patients with mild to moderate renal or hepatic impairment for rucaparib [52, 53] but the use of rucaparib in patients with severe renal or hepatic impairment has not been studied [55].

The coadministration of food or high-fat meal does not have clinically significant impact on pharmacokinetics, thus PARPis can be taken with or without food [21, 47, 48, 51, 54, 55].

Based on *in vitro* studies evidence, the concomitant use of strong or moderate CYP3A inhibitors or inducers with olaparib is not recommended [21, 51]. If the concomitant use of a CYP3A inhibitor cannot be avoided, olaparib dose shall be dose reduced [51]. Although no dose adjustment is needed for rucaparib, caution is recommended for concomitant administration with strong CYP3A and P-glycoprotein (P-gp) inhibitors [54, 55]. In contrast, niraparib is metabolized via carboxylesterases (CEs) catalyzed amide hydrolysis instead of CYP3A enzymes. There is low likelihood of clinically relevant interactions with other drugs and no dose adjustment is required [47, 48].

3.2 Adverse events associated with PARPis and management

The adverse events of PARPi are largely class effects and are well-characterized. The following section describes the most frequently observed adverse events in PARPi as a class, health care professionals (HCP) should always refer to the latest prescribing information or product information for further adverse event-related recommendations.

3.2.1 Fatigue

Fatigue/asthenia of any grade is one of the most common class-wide adverse events of PARPis reported in 50–70% of patients in various treatment settings. Dose interruption or dose reduction may be utilized to manage fatigue/asthenia symptoms in 3–13% of patients

[21, 44, 47, 48, 51, 54, 55]. Fatigue adverse events are largely mild to moderate (grade 1–2) and tend to occur early during initial phase of the PARPi therapy [56, 57].

It is important to note that patients may have baseline cancer-related fatigue as it affects 65% of patients with cancer [58]. Fatigue from chemotherapy can impact patient's desire to start maintenance therapy. Prior to the initiation of PARPi, HCPs shall assess and screen patient for baseline fatigue and counsel patient on the risks of fatigue as an adverse event of PARPi for shared treatment decision-making [59].

Fatigue can be scored and routinely assessed as a self-report subjective score using a 10-point numerical rating scale. Pharmacological treatment of psychostimulants may be considered for a short period after thorough evaluation. Physical exercises such as walking, aerobic, and resistance exercises are recommended in non-cachectic patients. Other modalities to manage fatigue include psychoeducation to help patients by promoting self-management, adaptation, and adjustment to their existing situation and environment, and cognitive behavioral therapy. Practicing mindfulness and yoga could be an option to improve fatigue symptoms [58, 59].

3.2.2 Gastrointestinal toxicities

Gastrointestinal toxicities of nausea, vomiting, and diarrhea are frequently reported with PARPi as a class-wide adverse events.

Nausea and vomiting were reported in 53–77% and 22–40% of patients, respectively [21, 44, 47, 48, 51, 54, 55]. Nausea and vomiting were generally reported early, with the first onset within the first few months of PARPi treatment [48, 57]. Both nausea and vomiting were generally low grade (grade 1 or 2) and can be managed by dose interruption and/or dose reduction in majority of patients [21, 44, 47, 48, 51, 54, 55].

Olaparib, niraparib, and rucaparib are categorized as moderate to high emetic risks (≥30% frequency of emesis) per National Comprehensive Cancer Network® (NCCN) antiemesis guideline v2.022. While chemotherapy-induced nausea and vomiting (CINV) may seem transient, it can cause a negative impact on patient's quality of life [60]. HCPs should assess patients who are at increased risk for CINV and counsel patients proactively. Risk factors of CINV include younger age, female sex, previous history of CINV, little or no previous alcohol use, prone to motion sickness, history of morning sickness during pregnancy, and anxiety/high pretreatment expectation of nausea. The use of single-agent prophylaxis with 5-HT3 reception agonists; granisetron, ondansetron, or dolasetron is recommended for prevention of emesis. Lorazepam may be added with or without histamine-2 blocker or proton pump inhibitor [61]. Bedtime administration of PARPi may be a potential method for managing nausea [47].

Diarrhea frequently occurred in 18–37% of patients. Grade ≥ 3 was infrequent, observed in ≤3% of patients [21, 44, 47, 48, 51, 54, 55]. For patients with mild to moderate diarrhea (grade 1–2), symptoms can be managed by oral hydration, dietary modification to avoid all lactose-containing products, high-osmolar dietary supplements, and the use of loperamide [62].

3.2.3 Hematologic toxicity

Hematologic toxicity (or myelosuppression) is a commonly recognized class-effect adverse event of PARPi that is linked to its mechanism of PARP trapping, which appears to drive cytotoxicity in healthy human bone marrow [56, 63]. Emerging clinical data suggest an inverse relationship between PARPi trapping potency and risks of myelosuppression adverse events [63]. Myelosuppression adverse events tend to occur in the early phase of PARPi maintenance treatment with median time to onset ranging from 22 to 80 days (~first 3 treatment cycles) [21, 48, 55, 64]. Although, grade ≥ 3 hematological adverse events tend to have a later onset [21, 55].

Anemia of any grade has been reported in 34–64% of patients receiving PARPi with grade ≥ 3 observed in 20–30% of patients. Permanently discontinuation due to anemia of PARPi was seen in ≤4% of patients in clinical trials [44, 47, 51, 54]. Neutropenia of any grade has been reported in 17–42% of patients receiving PARPi, neutropenia ≥ grade 3 was observed in less than ~20% of patients [44, 47, 51, 54]. Dose interruption or reduction may be used to manage anemia or neutropenia adverse events. For patients whose hemoglobin level falls <8 g/dL or if neutrophil count is <1000/mcL, PARPi should be held for a maximum of 28 days and blood counts or neutrophil counts to be monitored weekly until it returns to ≥9 g/dL or ≥ 1500/mcL, respectively. PARPi therapy may be resumed at a reduced dose [47].

Thrombocytopenia of any grade has been reported in ~10–30% of patients with a higher incidence of ~50–65% seen in patient receiving niraparib therapy [42, 45, 49, 52]. Grade ≥ 3 thrombocytopenia was more common in niraparib ranging from 20–30% compared to olaparib and rucaparib at 1–7% [44, 47, 51, 54]. For platelet count <100,000/mcL, niraparib can be held for a maximum of 28 days, platelet counts to be monitored weekly until recovery to ≥100,000/mcL. Niraparib may be resumed at the same or reduced dose but if platelet count was <75,000/mcL at the onset of adverse event occurrence, a reduced dose is recommended. If a patient experiences severe thrombocytopenia with a platelet count ≤10,000/mcL or if a patients has other risk factors of anticoagulation or antiplatelet drug use, these drugs should be held, and a platelet transfusion may be considered [47].

Overall, higher incidences of hematologic toxicity have been observed with niraparib, which is consistent with its pharmacologic properties as niraparib has higher PARP trapping potency relative to olaparib and rucaparib [65, 66]. As discussed above in Section 2.2, individualized starting dose of niraparib was evaluated prospectively in 35% of patients in the PRIMA trial. Results showed improved safety and tolerability of niraparib [42].

3.2.4 Off-target effects

Hypertension and hypertensive crisis have been reported among patients who were treated with niraparib. Grade ≥ 3 hypertension occurred in 5–9% of patients across treatment settings. Niraparib's pharmacological inhibition of the dopamine transporter, norepinephrine transporter, and serotonin transporter, demonstrated in an *in vitro* pharmacology screen may explain its unique effects on pulse rate and blood pressure. As such, blood pressure and heart rate monitoring weekly for the first 2 months, then monthly for the first year of treatment, and periodically thereafter is recommended [47, 48].

Posterior reversible encephalopathy syndrome (PRES) is a rare, reversible, neurological disorder that presents with symptoms including seizure, headache, altered mental status, visual disturbance, or cortical blindness, with or without associated hypertension. PRES was observed in 0.1% of 2165 patients treated with niraparib in clinical trials and post-marketing reports. If PRES is suspected, discontinue niraparib and specific symptoms associated with PRES shall be treated [47, 48].

3.2.5 Myelodysplastic syndrome (MDS)/acute myeloid leukemia (AML)

MDS/AML occurred in patients treated with PARPi with incidences ranging from 0.2%–1.7% in ovarian cancer clinical trials setting and some cases were fatal [21, 44, 47, 48, 51, 54, 55]. In a pharmacovigilance analysis of the FDA Adverse Events Reporting System (FAERS) database, a total of 319 cases of PARPi-associated MDS/AML were identified from the period of quarter (Q)4, 2014 to Q1, 2020. Death or other life-threatening outcomes were reported in 49% of cases [67]. The duration of PARPi treatment varied from 1 month to >10 years. In all cases, patients had received previous platinum-based chemotherapy and/or other DNA damaging agents including radiation [21, 44, 47, 48, 51, 54, 55].

The mechanism of PARPi associated with MDS/AML remains unclear [67]. It is recommended to not start PARPi therapy until patients have recovered from hematological toxicity caused by prior chemotherapy (≤ grade 1). For prolonged hematologic toxicities >4 weeks, patient shall be referred to a hematologist for further evaluation. If MDS/AML is confirmed, discontinue PARPi permanently [21, 44, 47, 48, 51, 55].

4. General recommendations for patient selection for front-line maintenance PARPi treatment

For decades the initial therapeutic approach for patients with EOC relied on surgery followed by platinum-based chemotherapy [68]. Surgery allows confirmation of the diagnosis, as well as staging of the disease. The main goal of the primary debulking surgery (PDS), which plays a cardinal role in the overall management of advanced EOC (stages III and IV), is to obtain an optimal cytoreduction defined as complete resection of all visible tumors [69]. When complete cytoreduction is not attainable, either due to an extensive disease burden or to poor performance status, the patients are treated first with neoadjuvant platinum-based chemotherapy [70, 71]. This strategy usually encompasses the administration of three cycles of chemotherapy and upon response to the systemic treatment, the interval debulking surgery (IDS) is performed. After surgery, chemotherapy is continued for up to six cycles. When PDS is considered appropriate, intravenous platinum and taxane regimen every 21 days for six cycles represent the adjuvant treatment [72]. However, the timing of surgical intervention in relation to systemic treatment (neoadjuvant vs. adjuvant) is still an unsettled matter.

Since 2011, in the first line setting, the addition of the vascular endothelial growth factor inhibitor (VEGFi), bevacizumab to chemotherapy following debulking surgery has become SOC given the positive results relative to PFS benefit demonstrated in two randomized phase III trials, GOG-0218 and ICON7 [49, 50]. However, the addition of bevacizumab is currently recommended in a subgroup of patients with poor prognosis, namely patients with stage III and residual disease after surgery or stage IV based on a post hoc overall survival analysis.

With the advent of PARPis in the clinic, the paradigm for the treatment of EOC has undergone remarkable changes. To assist health care providers, clinical practice guidelines have been updated to support the decision-making process and to ensure consistency of treatment is aligned with current best evidence-based medicine. In addition to this practice, we also strongly advocate as a primary principle, that sound clinical judgment (e.g., concern relative to treatment-associated toxicity, performance status, and other comorbidities) and patient preference should be also considered. This mindset is extremely important especially when the risk-benefit profile of treatment in a subset of patients has not been clearly established and, therefore, other management options are available.

For newly diagnosed patients, testing for BRCA mutation (germline/somatic) is strongly recommended, given that systemic therapeutic options are available in frontline setting. Maintenance use of olaparib for 2 years as first-line management approach should be the SOC for all patients with BRCA1/2 mutation in newly diagnosed advanced EOC after a response to chemotherapy based on SOLO-1 trial results. As mentioned in the 5-year follow-up analysis of SOLO-1, olaparib recipients had doubled the median PFS compared to those treated with placebo [46].

If BRCA mutation (germline/somatic) results are negative, HRD test should be considered to identify a subgroup of women who are BRCA wild type but derive greater clinical benefit from a PARPi. In the presence of positive HRD score after CR or PR to front-line platinum-based chemotherapy, maintenance use of niraparib for 3 years or olaparib in combination with bevacizumab are available options based on PRIMA and PAOLA-1 study, respectively. Both studies enrolled newly diagnosed EOC patients, regardless of their BRCA status.

PRIMA trial enrolled high-risk patients, that is, 35% of patients had stage IV [42] and 45% of patients had visible disease after PDS or IDS [73]. Among patients with HRD and BRCA wild type, the median PFS was 19.6 months in the niraparib group vs. 8.2 months in the placebo group (HR = 0.50; 95% CI 0.31–0.83) [42].

In PAOLA-1 trial, the median PFS was 28.1 months vs. 16.6 months, respectively, for HRD-positive BRCA wild-type. Due to that fact that PAOLA-1 study design did not have olaparib maintenance only arm, the value of adding bevacizumab remains uncertain [41].

Patients with HRR-proficient tumors have poorer prognosis. Nonetheless, for woman whose tumor is found to be HRR proficient (HRD negative), PARPi monotherapy can still be offered, despite the diminished clinical benefit seen among this cohort of women based on PRIMA trial results. [74] In HRD-negative patients, niraparib demonstrated a modest yet statistically significant improvement in median PFS 8.1 months vs. 5.4 months, with niraparib versus placebo (HR 0.68, CI 95% 0.49–0.94). Conversely, in PAOLA-1 study, olaparib plus bevacizumab did not show a significant improvement in PFS in HRD-negative patients [41].

Therefore, bevacizumab monotherapy regimen upfront after induction with chemotherapy may be considered a valid strategy in patients with HRD negative tumors considering specific clinical characteristics (e.g., pleural effusions or ascites) with the option to administer a PARPi in later lines upon recurrence. It has been noted, however, that this approach will need to demonstrate a subsequent response to platinum to guarantee PARPis sensitivity. Indeed, the American Society of Clinical Oncology (ASCO) guideline supports the use of PARPis in all patients with advanced EOC in the front-line maintenance setting regardless of HRD status. Based on the current label, only niraparib is approved in the first-line maintenance treatment setting regardless of biomarker status. In this scenario, bevacizumab could be postponed to later line for the treatment of women with both platinum-sensitive and platinum-resistant diseases [75].

Lastly, given that patients enrolled in these studies excluded women who previously received PARPi, no data are currently available on the efficacy of retreatment with PARPi after progression. Hence, up to this point, the recommendation advises against PARP inhibitor retreatment in advance EOC [75]. Needless to say, this area of research is becoming the highest unmet need in ovarian cancer due to the increasing patient population receiving first-line PARPis.

5. Conclusion

The main objective of this chapter was to highlight the recent contribution brought by the approval of PARPis for the treatment of advanced EOC. The PARPis clinical development underscored the value of the "bench to bedside framework" which translates basic biological knowledge into medical therapeutic application.

Initially developed as maintenance therapy in patients with complete or partial response after platinum-based chemotherapy in a recurrent setting, PARPi is now approved in multiple settings including as a frontline management strategy. However, the use of these novel agents early in the disease trajectory exposes new therapeutic challenges associated with PARPi-resistance which clinically leads to treatment failure. As a result, uncovering the molecular mechanisms linked to acquired and intrinsic resistance to PARPi is an active area of research. Overall increased drug efflux (which leads to reduced intracellular drug concentrations), restoration of HRR repair (re-expression of functional proteins involved in HRR or somatic reversion mutations in either *BRCA1* or *BRCA2*), and aberrations in PARP signaling are the common pathways involved in PARPi resistance [76]. A detailed elucidation of these molecular events would be essential for the design of new therapeutic strategies to prevent/overcome resistance. Currently, several hypotheses within clinical trials (targeted combination intervention) are under investigation with the aim to re-sensitize and enhance ovarian cancer cells to PARPis, while optimizing tolerability and quality of life. The hope is that there will be a continuous improvement in targeted therapies leading to an extension of overall survival and an effective curability of this disease.

Conflict of interest

Nicola Di Santo is employed by Pfizer, Inc. and has an ownership interest (including stocks); Yin Wong is employed by GSK, plc and has an ownership interest (including stocks).

Author details

Nicola Di Santo[1*], Greta Bagnolini[2], Yin Wong[3], Marco Carnelli[1] and Luigi Frigerio[4]

1 Department Obstetrics and Gynecology, Papa Giovanni XXIII, Bergamo, Italy

2 Duke University, Durham, North Carolina, United States

3 GSK plc., Waltham, Massachusetts, United States

4 Department Obstetrics and Gynecology, Policlinico San Pietro—Università Vita e Salute, Bergamo, Italy

*Address all correspondence to: niconcus@gmail.com

References

[1] Sung H, Ferlay J, Siegel RL, Laversanne M, Soerjomataram I, Jemal A, et al. Global cancer statistics 2020: GLOBOCAN estimates of incidence and mortality worldwide for 36 cancers in 185 countries. CA: A Cancer Journal for Clinicians. 2021; **71**(3):209-249

[2] Goff BA, Mandel LS, Melancon CH, Muntz HG. Frequency of symptoms of ovarian cancer in women presenting to primary care clinics. Journal of the American Medical Association. 2004; **291**(22):2705-2712

[3] Jacobs IJ, Menon U, Ryan A, Gentry-Maharaj A, Burnell M, Kalsi JK, et al. Ovarian cancer screening and mortality in the UK collaborative trial of ovarian cancer screening (UKCTOCS): A randomised controlled trial. Lancet. 2016;**387**(10022):945-956

[4] Labidi-Galy SI, Papp E, Hallberg D, Niknafs N, Adleff V, Noe M, et al. High grade serous ovarian carcinomas originate in the fallopian tube. Nature Communications. 2017;**8**(1):1093

[5] Ducie J, Dao F, Considine M, Olvera N, Shaw PA, Kurman RJ, et al. Molecular analysis of high-grade serous ovarian carcinoma with and without associated serous tubal intra-epithelial carcinoma. Nature Communications. 2017;**8**(1):990

[6] Cancer Genome Atlas Research N. integrated genomic analyses of ovarian carcinoma. Nature. 2011;**474**(7353): 609-615

[7] Kuchenbaecker KB, Hopper JL, Barnes DR, Phillips KA, Mooij TM, Roos-Blom MJ, et al. Risks of breast, ovarian, and contralateral breast cancer for BRCA1 and BRCA2 mutation carriers. Journal of the American Medical Association. 2017;**317**(23):2402-2416

[8] McCabe N, Turner NC, Lord CJ, Kluzek K, Bialkowska A, Swift S, et al. Deficiency in the repair of DNA damage by homologous recombination and sensitivity to poly(ADP-ribose) polymerase inhibition. Cancer Research. 2006;**66**(16):8109-8115

[9] Langelier MF, Eisemann T, Riccio AA, Pascal JM. PARP family enzymes: Regulation and catalysis of the poly(ADP-ribose) posttranslational modification. Current Opinion in Structural Biology. 2018;**53**:187-198

[10] Ray Chaudhuri A, Nussenzweig A. The multifaceted roles of PARP1 in DNA repair and chromatin remodelling. Nature Reviews. Molecular Cell Biology. 2017;**18**(10):610-621

[11] Eleazer R, Fondufe-Mittendorf YN. The multifaceted role of PARP1 in RNA biogenesis. Wiley Interdisciplinary Review RNA. 2021;**12**(2):e1617

[12] Kim DS, Camacho CV, Kraus WL. Alternate therapeutic pathways for PARP inhibitors and potential mechanisms of resistance. Experimental & Molecular Medicine. 2021;**53**(1):42-51

[13] Eustermann S, Wu WF, Langelier MF, Yang JC, Easton LE, Riccio AA, et al. Structural basis of detection and signaling of DNA single-strand breaks by human PARP-1. Molecular Cell. 2015;**60**(5):742-754

[14] Lord CJ, Ashworth A. PARP inhibitors: Synthetic lethality in the clinic. Science. 2017;**355**(6330):1152-1158

[15] El-Khamisy SF, Masutani M, Suzuki H, Caldecott KW. A requirement

for PARP-1 for the assembly or stability of XRCC1 nuclear foci at sites of oxidative DNA damage. Nucleic Acids Research. 2003;**31**(19):5526-5533

[16] Zhu H, Wei M, Xu J, Hua J, Liang C, Meng Q, et al. PARP inhibitors in pancreatic cancer: Molecular mechanisms and clinical applications. Molecular Cancer. 2020;**19**(1):49

[17] Alemasova EE, Pestryakov PE, Sukhanova MV, Kretov DA, Moor NA, Curmi PA, et al. Poly(ADP-ribosyl)ation as a new posttranslational modification of YB-1. Biochimie. 2015;**119**:36-44

[18] Dziadkowiec KN, Gasiorowska E, Nowak-Markwitz E, Jankowska A. PARP inhibitors: Review of mechanisms of action and BRCA1/2 mutation targeting. Prz Menopauzalny. 2016;**15**(4):215-219

[19] Krastev DB, Wicks AJ, Lord CJ. PARP inhibitors - trapped in a toxic love affair. Cancer Research. 2021;**81**(22): 5605-5607

[20] Lord CJ, Ashworth A. BRCAness revisited. Nature Reviews. Cancer. 2016; **16**(2):110-120

[21] Lynparza (olaparib) [European Public Assessment Report: Product Information]. European Medicines Agency; 2022. Available from: https://www.ema.europa.eu/documents/product-information/lynparza-epar-product-information_en.pdf

[22] Fong PC, Boss DS, Yap TA, Tutt A, Wu P, Mergui-Roelvink M, et al. Inhibition of poly(ADP-ribose) polymerase in tumors from BRCA mutation carriers. The New England Journal of Medicine. 2009;**361**(2): 123-134

[23] Ledermann J, Harter P, Gourley C, Friedlander M, Vergote I, Rustin G, et al. Olaparib maintenance therapy in platinum-sensitive relapsed ovarian cancer. The New England Journal of Medicine. 2012;**366**(15):1382-1392

[24] Ledermann J, Harter P, Gourley C, Friedlander M, Vergote I, Rustin G, et al. Olaparib maintenance therapy in patients with platinum-sensitive relapsed serous ovarian cancer: A preplanned retrospective analysis of outcomes by BRCA status in a randomised phase 2 trial. The Lancet Oncology. 2014;**15**(8):852-861

[25] LYNPARZA® (olaparib) capsules [package insert]. Wilmington (DE): AstraZeneca Pharmaceuticals LP; 2017. Available from: https://www.accessdata.fda.gov/drugsatfda_docs/label/2017/208558s000lbl.pdf

[26] Pujade-Lauraine E, Ledermann JA, Selle F, Gebski V, Penson RT, Oza AM, et al. Olaparib tablets as maintenance therapy in patients with platinum-sensitive, relapsed ovarian cancer and a BRCA1/2 mutation (SOLO2/ENGOT-Ov21): A double-blind, randomised, placebo-controlled, phase 3 trial. The Lancet Oncology. 2017;**18**(9):1274-1284

[27] ZEJULA® (niraparib) capsules [package insert]. Waltham (MA); 2017. Available from: https://www.accessdata.fda.gov/drugsatfda_docs/label/2017/208447lbl.pdf

[28] Mirza MR, Monk BJ, Herrstedt J, Oza AM, Mahner S, Redondo A, et al. Niraparib maintenance therapy in platinum-sensitive, recurrent ovarian Cancer. The New England Journal of Medicine. 2016;**375**(22):2154-2164

[29] RUBRACA® (rucaparib) tablets [Multi=Discipline Review/Summary, Clinical, Non-Clinical]. Food and Drug Administration; 2016. Available from: https://www.accessdata.fda.gov/drugsa

tfda_docs/nda/2016/209115Orig1s000MultiDisciplineR.pdf

[30] Coleman RL, Oza AM, Lorusso D, Aghajanian C, Oaknin A, Dean A, et al. Rucaparib maintenance treatment for recurrent ovarian carcinoma after response to platinum therapy (ARIEL3): A randomised, double-blind, placebo-controlled, phase 3 trial. Lancet. 2017; **390**(10106):1949-1961

[31] Kim G, Ison G, McKee AE, Zhang H, Tang S, Gwise T, et al. FDA approval summary: Olaparib monotherapy in patients with deleterious germline BRCA-mutated advanced ovarian cancer treated with three or more lines of chemotherapy. Clinical Cancer Research. 2015;**21**(19):4257-4261

[32] Kaufman B, Shapira-Frommer R, Schmutzler RK, Audeh MW, Friedlander M, Balmana J, et al. Olaparib monotherapy in patients with advanced cancer and a germline BRCA1/2 mutation. Journal of Clinical Oncology. 2015;**33**(3):244-250

[33] Penson RT, Valencia RV, Cibula D, Colombo N, Leath CA 3rd, Bidzinski M, et al. Olaparib versus nonplatinum chemotherapy in patients with platinum-sensitive relapsed ovarian cancer and a germline BRCA1/2 mutation (SOLO3): A randomized phase III trial. Journal of Clinical Oncology. 2020;**38**(11):1164-1174

[34] LYNPARZA® (olaparib) tablets [important prescribing information]. Wilmington (DE): AstraZeneca Pharmaceuticals LP; 2022. Available from: https://www.lynparzahcp.com/content/dam/physician-services/us/590-lynparza-hcp-branded/hcp-global/pdf/solo3-dhcp-final-signed.pdf

[35] Swisher EM, Lin KK, Oza AM, Scott CL, Giordano H, Sun J, et al. Rucaparib in relapsed, platinum-sensitive high-grade ovarian carcinoma (ARIEL2 Part 1): An international, multicentre, open-label, phase 2 trial. The Lancet Oncology. 2017;**18**(1):75-87

[36] Balasubramaniam S, Beaver JA, Horton S, Fernandes LL, Tang S, Horne HN, et al. FDA approval summary: Rucaparib for the treatment of patients with deleterious BRCA mutation-associated advanced ovarian cancer. Clinical Cancer Research. 2017; **23**(23):7165-7170

[37] Kristeleit R, Lisyanskaya A, Fedenko A, Dvokin M, de Melo AC, Sharyk Y, et al. Rucaparib versus standard-of-care chemotherapy in patients with relapsed ovarian cancer and a deleterious BRCA1 or BRCA2 mutation (ARIEL4): An international, open-label, randomised, phase 3 trial. The Lancet Oncology. 2022;**23**(4): 465-478

[38] RUBRACA® (Rucaparib) Tablets [Important Prescribing Information]. Boulder (CO): Clovis Oncology, Inc.; 2022. Available from: https://clovisoncology.com/pdfs/US_DHCPL_final_signed.pdf

[39] Moore KN, Secord AA, Geller MA, Miller DS, Cloven N, Fleming GF, et al. Niraparib monotherapy for late-line treatment of ovarian cancer (QUADRA): A multicentre, open-label, single-arm, phase 2 trial. The Lancet Oncology. 2019; **20**(5):636-648

[40] Moore K, Colombo N, Scambia G, Kim BG, Oaknin A, Friedlander M, et al. Maintenance Olaparib in patients with newly diagnosed advanced ovarian Cancer. The New England Journal of Medicine. 2018;**379**(26):2495-2505

[41] Ray-Coquard I, Pautier P, Pignata S, Perol D, Gonzalez-Martin A, Berger R,

et al. Olaparib plus bevacizumab as first-line maintenance in ovarian cancer. The New England Journal of Medicine. 2019; **381**(25):2416-2428

[42] González-Martín A, Pothuri B, Vergote I, DePont CR, Graybill W, Mirza MR, et al. Niraparib in patients with newly diagnosed advanced ovarian cancer. New England Journal of Medicine. 2019;**381**(25):2391-2402

[43] Coleman RL, Fleming GF, Brady MF, Swisher EM, Steffensen KD, Friedlander M, et al. Veliparib with first-line chemotherapy and as maintenance therapy in ovarian cancer. The New England Journal of Medicine. 2019; **381**(25):2403-2415

[44] Monk BJ, Parkinson C, Lim MC, O'Malley DM, Oaknin A,Wilson MK, Coleman RL, et al. Phase III trial to evaluate rucaparib monotherapy as maintenance treatment in patients with newly diagnosed ovarian cancer. Journal of Clinical Oncology. 2022;**2022:** JCO2201003

[45] LYNPARZA® (olaparib) tablets [package insert]. Wilmington (DE): AstraZeneca Pharmaceuticals LP; 2018. Available from: https://www.accessdata.fda.gov/drugsatfda_docs/label/2018/208558s006lbl.pdf

[46] Banerjee SM, Colombo N, Scambia G, Kim BG, Oaknin A, Friedlander M, et al. Maintenance olaparib for patients (pts) with newly diagnosed, advanced ovarian cancer (OC) and a BRCA mutation (BRCAm): 5-year (y) follow-up (f/u) from SOLO1. Annals of Oncology. 2020;**31:** S551-SA89

[47] ZEJULA (Niraparib) Capsules [Package Insert]. Research Triangle Park (NC): GlaxoSmithKline; 2022. Available from: https://gskpro.com/content/dam/global/hcpportal/en_US/Prescribing_Information/Zejula_Capsules/pdf/ZEJULA-CAPSULES-PI-PIL.PDF

[48] Zejula (niraparib) [European Public Assessment Report: Product Information]. European Medicines Agency; 2022. Available from: https://www.ema.europa.eu/documents/product-information/zejula-epar-product-information_en.pdf

[49] Burger RA, Brady MF, Bookman MA, Fleming GF, Monk BJ, Huang H, et al. Incorporation of bevacizumab in the primary treatment of ovarian cancer. The New England Journal of Medicine. 2011;**365**(26): 2473-2483

[50] Perren TJ, Swart AM, Pfisterer J, Ledermann JA, Pujade-Lauraine E, Kristensen G, et al. A phase 3 trial of bevacizumab in ovarian cancer. The New England Journal of Medicine. 2011; **365**(26):2484-2496

[51] LYNPARZA® (olaparib) tablets [package insert]. Wilmington (DE): AstraZeneca Pharmaceuticals LP; 2022. Available from: http://www.azpicentral.com/pi.html?product=lynparza_tb

[52] Kaye SB, Lubinski J, Matulonis U, Ang JE, Gourley C, Karlan BY, et al. Phase II, open-label, randomized, multicenter study comparing the efficacy and safety of olaparib, a poly (ADP-ribose) polymerase inhibitor, and pegylated liposomal doxorubicin in patients with BRCA1 or BRCA2 mutations and recurrent ovarian cancer. Journal of Clinical Oncology. 2012;**30**(4): 372-379

[53] Donawho CK, Luo Y, Luo Y, Penning TD, Bauch JL, Bouska JJ, et al. ABT-888, an orally active poly (ADP-ribose) polymerase inhibitor that potentiates DNA-damaging agents in

preclinical tumor models. Clinical Cancer Research. 2007;**13**(9):2728-2737

[54] RUBRACA® (Rucaparib) Tablets [Package Insert]. Boulder (CO): Clovis Oncology, Inc.; 2022. Available from: https://clovisoncology.com/pdfs/RubracaUSPI.pdf

[55] Rubraca (rucaparib) [European Public Assessment Report: Product Information]. European Medicines Agency; 2022. Available from: https://www.ema.europa.eu/documents/product-information/rubraca-epar-product-information_en.pdf

[56] Madariaga A, Bowering V, Ahrari S, Oza AM, Lheureux S. Manage wisely: Poly (ADP-ribose) polymerase inhibitor (PARPI) treatment and adverse events. International Journal of Gynecologic Cancer. 2020;**30**(7):903-915

[57] Oza AM, Matulonis UA, Malander S, et al. Quality of life in patients with recurrent ovarian cancer treated with niraparib versus placebo (ENGOT-OV16/NOVA): Results from a double-blind, phase 3, randomised controlled trial. The Lancet Oncology. 2018;**19**: 1117-1125

[58] Fabi A, Bhargava R, Fatigoni S, Guglielmo M, Horneber M, Roila F, et al. Cancer-related fatigue: ESMO clinical practice guidelines for diagnosis and treatment. Annals of Oncology. 2020; **31**(6):713-723

[59] Moore KN, Monk BJ. Patient counseling and management of symptoms during Olaparib therapy for recurrent ovarian cancer. The Oncologist. 2016;**21**(8):954-963

[60] Yeo W, Mo FKF, Yip CCH, Yeo VA, Li L, Lau TKH, et al. Quality of life associated with nausea and vomiting from anthracycline-based chemotherapy: A pooled data analysis from three prospective trials. The Oncologist. 2021;**26**(12):e2288-e2e96

[61] National Comprehensive Cancer Network (NCCN). NCCN clinical practice guidelines in oncology. Antiemesis. Version 2, 2022. Available from: https://www.nccn.org/professionals/physician_gls/pdf/antiemesis.pdf

[62] Bossi P, Antonuzzo A, Cherny NI, Rosengarten O, Pernot S, Trippa F, et al. Diarrhoea in adult cancer patients: ESMO Clinical Practice Guidelines. Annals of Oncology. 2018;**29**:iv126-iiv42

[63] Hopkins TA, Ainsworth WB, Ellis PA, Donawho CK, DiGiammarino EL, Panchal SC, et al. PARP1 trapping by PARP inhibitors drives cytotoxicity in both cancer cells and healthy bone marrow. Molecular Cancer Research. 2019;**17**(2):409-419

[64] Berek JS, Matulonis UA, Peen U, Ghatage P, Mahner S, Redondo A, et al. Safety and dose modification for patients receiving niraparib. Annals of Oncology. 2018;**29**(8):1784-1792

[65] Murai J, Huang SY, Renaud A, Zhang Y, Ji J, Takeda S, et al. Stereospecific PARP trapping by BMN 673 and comparison with olaparib and rucaparib. Molecular Cancer Therapeutics. 2014;**13**(2):433-443

[66] Murai J, Huang SY, Das BB, Renaud A, Zhang Y, Doroshow JH, et al. Trapping of PARP1 and PARP2 by clinical PARP inhibitors. Cancer Research. 2012;**72**(21):5588-5599

[67] Ma Z, Sun XM, Lu WC, Zhao ZX, Xu ZM, Lyu JY, et al. Poly(ADP-ribose) polymerase inhibitor-associated myelodysplastic syndrome/acute myeloid leukemia: A pharmacovigilance

analysis of the FAERS database. ESMO Open. 2021;**6**(1):100033

[68] Griffiths CT, Fuller AF. Intensive surgical and chemotherapeutic management of advanced ovarian cancer. The Surgical Clinics of North America. 1978;**58**(1):131-142

[69] Chang SJ, Hodeib M, Chang J, Bristow RE. Survival impact of complete cytoreduction to no gross residual disease for advanced-stage ovarian cancer: A meta-analysis. Gynecologic Oncology. 2013;**130**:493-498

[70] Vergote I, Tropé CG, Amant F, et al. Neoadjuvant chemotherapy or primary surgery in stage IIIC or IV ovarian cancer. The New England Journal of Medicine. 2010;**363**:943-953

[71] Kehoe A, Hook J, Nankivell M, et al. Primary chemotherapy versus primary surgery for newly diagnosed advanced ovarian cancer (CHORUS): An open-label, randomised, controlled, non-inferiority trial. Lancet. 2015;**386**: 249-257

[72] Ozols RF, Bundy BN, Greer BE, et al. Phase III trial of carboplatin and paclitaxel compared with cisplatin and paclitaxel in patients with optimally resected stage III ovarian cancer: A Gynecologic oncology group study. Journal of Clinical Oncology. 2003;**21**:3194

[73] O'Cearbhaill RE, Perez-Fidalgo JA, Monk BJ, Tusquets I, McCormick C, Fuentes J, et al. Efficacy of niraparib by time of surgery and postoperative residual disease status: A post hoc analysis of patients in the PRIMA/ENGOT-OV26/GOG-3012 study. Gynaecology and Oncology. 2022; **166**(1):36-43

[74] Banerjee S, Gonzalez-Martin A, Harter P, Lorusso D, Moore KN, Oaknin A, et al. First-line PARP inhibitors in ovarian cancer: Summary of an ESMO open - cancer horizons round-table discussion. ESMO Open [Internet]. 2020;**5**(6)

[75] Tew WP, Lacchetti C, Ellis A, Maxian K, Banerjee S, Bookman M, et al. PARP inhibitors in the management of ovarian cancer: ASCO guideline. Journal of Clinical Oncology. 2020;**38**(30): 3468-3493

[76] D'Andrea AD. Mechanisms of PARP inhibitor sensitivity and resistance. DNA Repair. 2018;**2018**(71):172-176